Lynda AOUDIA

Imaging osteoarthropathies of endocrine origin

Lynda AOUDIA

Imaging osteoarthropathies of endocrine origin

ScienciaScripts

Imprint

Cover image: www.ingimage.com

This book is a translation from the original published under ISBN 978-620-6-70425-6.

Publisher:
Sciencia Scripts
is a trademark of
Dodo Books Indian Ocean Ltd. and OmniScriptum S.R.L publishing group

120 High Road, East Finchley, London, N2 9ED, United Kingdom
Str. Armeneasca 28/1, office 1, Chisinau MD-2012, Republic of Moldova, Europe
Printed at: see last page
ISBN: 978-620-7-74323-0

Foreword

Bone tissue is constantly being remodeled under the control of hormonal factors. As a result, most endocrine disorders are accompanied by changes in the musculoskeletal system. In current radiological practice, the main osteoarticular complications encountered are those of post-menopausal osteoporosis, diabetes and hyperparathyroidism. Alterations secondary to acromegaly are less frequent, but it is important to be aware of them in order to make an early diagnosis. Dysthyroid changes are rare and unspecific.

The aim of this book is to explain the main radiological features of these endocrinopathies, so that diagnosis can be made as early as possible.

Prof. Lynda AOUDIA

Table of contents

Preface 1

Table of contents 2

Introduction 3

Endocrine system 4

1. Pituitary gland 5

2. Parathyroid 17

3. Thyroid 34

4. Adrenals 40

5. Pancreas 49

6. Gonads 60

References 65

Introduction

Osteoarticular manifestations accompanying endocrine disorders are now rare. Endocrinopathies have benefited from earlier diagnosis, thanks to advances in biology, and more effective treatment, often initiated early, before the development of bone manifestations. Most radiological descriptions of endocrine osteopathies are old, and few new imaging studies have been published, which explains why standard radiography is still the main method of exploration in this field.

Endocrine system

Many hormones are involved in the regulation of bone remodeling. Some have an anabolic effect on bone tissue, promoting the action of osteoblasts or inhibiting that of osteoclasts: growth hormone (GH) and insulin-like growth factor 1 (IGF1) [1], insulin [2] and sex steroids (adrenal and gonadal androgens and estrogens). Other hormones, on the other hand, promote bone resorption: parathyroid hormone (PTH), vitamin D, thyroid hormones (T3, T4) and glucocorticoids.

Most hormones regulate bone remodelling, which is why most endocrinopathies are accompanied by osteoarticular manifestations (fig. 1).

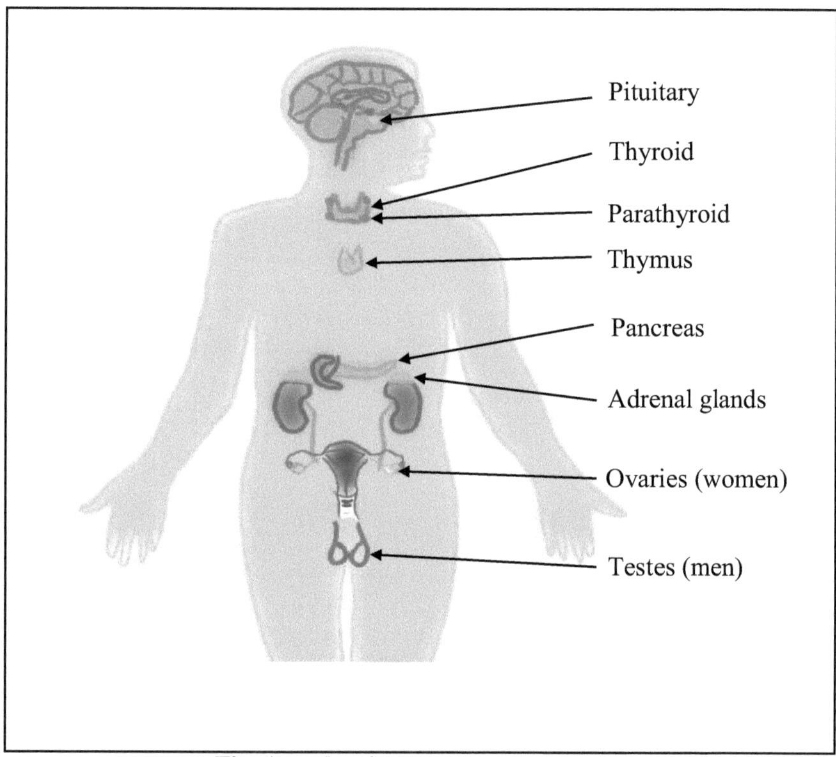

Fig. 1. endocrine system.

1. Pituitary gland

The anterior pituitary secretes GH (growth hormone) and regulates the hormonal secretion of numerous endocrine glands, such as the thyroid, adrenals and gonads. Its dysfunction is at the root of bone metabolism disorders, directly through abnormal GH secretion, and indirectly through dysregulation of the target glands.

1.1. Acromegaly

Acromegaly is the result of hypersecretion of GH, which stimulates cartilage and bone proliferation. In the vast majority of cases, GH excess is linked to a pituitary somatotropic cell adenoma.
Acromegaly is a rare disease, affecting 1 in 140,000 to 250,000 people, with the same incidence in both sexes [3].

1.1.1. Clinic

The disease develops slowly and tremulously, and is often diagnosed more than 10 years after the onset of hypersecretion [4].
Apart from pituitary tumor syndrome, such as headaches, visual disturbances, bitemporal hemianopsia and, more rarely, occulo-motor paralysis, it is often complications that reveal the pathology. Some of the clinical signs found in the disease are :

- Functional signs: asthenia, bone pain.
- Cutaneous signs: thickened skin, diffuse hypersudation.
- Metabolic and vascular repercussions: arterial hypertension, left ventricular hypertrophy and heart failure, glucose intolerance and even diabetes.
- Acromegaly increases the risk of cancer: thyroid, colon...[5].
-

1.1.2. Biology

GH levels are often elevated but may remain normal (although the nycthemeral cycle is disturbed). IGF1 levels are generally elevated. Dynamic tests confirm the diagnosis (braking to hyperglycemia, paradoxical GH response to thyrostimulin releasing hormone [TRH] injection).

1.1.3. Imaging

Magnetic resonance imaging (MRI) is used to study pituitary adenomas (fig. 2), while standard X-rays are generally sufficient to assess the skeletal changes associated with the disease (fig. 3).

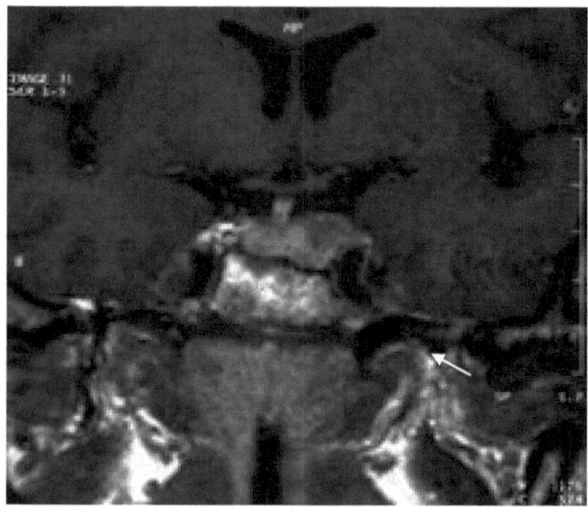

Fig. 2. Acromegaly. T1 sequence MRI after gadolinium injection, coronal slice Pituitary adenoma (arrow). The adenoma appears hyposignal in relation to the rest of the anteropituitary gland.

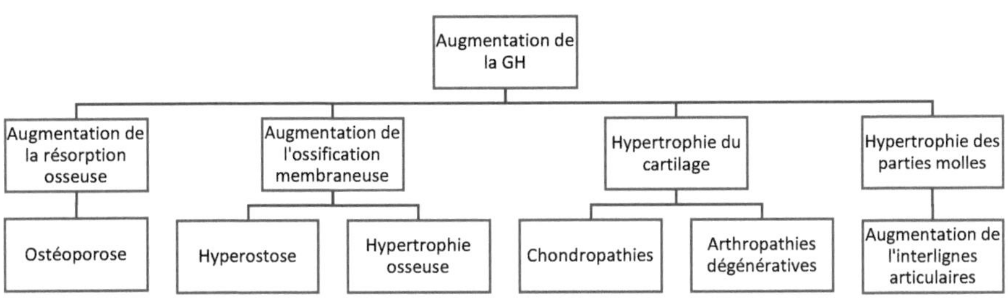

Fig. 3: Pathophysiology of bone changes in acromegaly [6].

1.1.3.1.Technical

In the case of acromegaly, bone manifestations warrant, as a minimum, the following standard radiographs:

- front hands and feet,
- dorsolumbar spine face and profile,
- skull in profile,
- front thorax.

Exploration of peripheral joints is guided by symptomatology.

1.1.3.2.Skull

On standard radiography, the following signs are found (fig. 4):

- Widening of the sella turcica.
- Hypertrophy of the cranial vault tables.
- Protrusion of orbital margins with hypertrophy of frontal sinuses.
- Hypertrophy of the external occipital protuberance.
- Enlargement of the mandible, responsible for prognathism and disorders of the dental articulation.

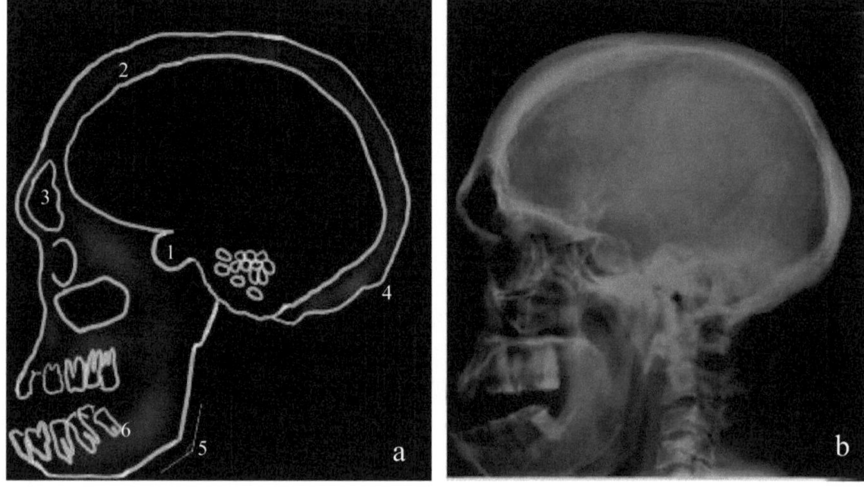

Fig. 4. Acromegaly. (a) Schematic diagram. (b) Standard skull radiograph in profile. 1. Ballooning of the sella turcica.

2. Thickening of the vault.
3. Hypertrophy of the frontal sinus.
4. Hypertrophy of the external occipital protuberance.
5. Opening of the jaw angle with prognathism.
6. Dental articulation disorders.

Plantar pad thickening greater than 22 mm

1.1.3.3.Hands and feet

At the onset of the disease, soft tissue hypertrophy is seen mainly in the plantar pad on a profile X-ray of the foot (fig. 5). Tissue thickening also affects cartilage and synovial tissue, resulting in significant widening of the joint spaces.

The appearance is very characteristic of the metacarpophalangeal (MCP) joints, especially the 2^e and 3^e MCPs on a frontal hand X-ray, and is often one of the first radiological manifestations of the disease [7] (fig. 6, 7). Signs found in the hand are as follows:

- Thickening of the soft parts of the hand.
- Widening of the metacarpophalangeal interlines.
- Hypertrophy of the bony ridges on the lateral surfaces of the metacarpals and phalanges.
- Deformed phalangeal tassels with anchor-like appearance.
- Increased distance between radial and ulnar styloids.

–

Fig. 5. Acromegaly. (a) Schematic diagram. (b) Standard profile foot X-ray.

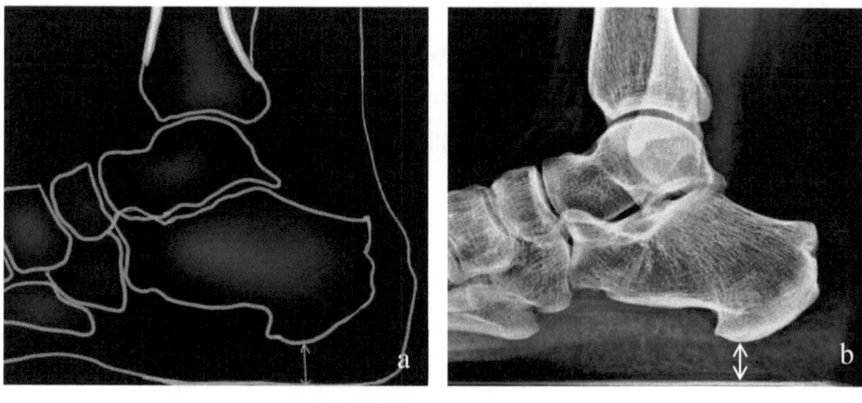

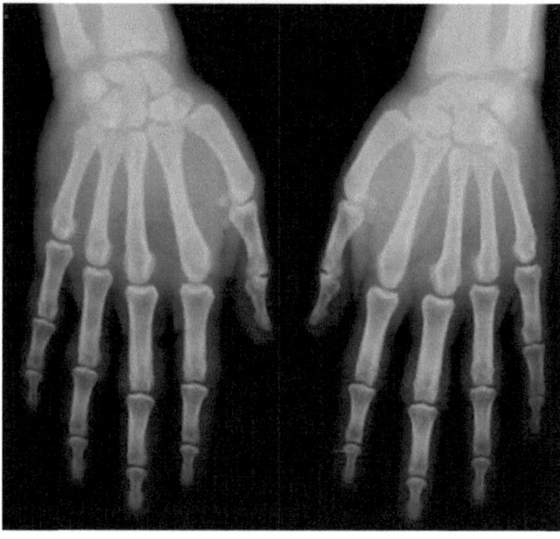

Fig. 6. Acromegaly. Front X-ray of the hands. Enlargement of the metacarpophalangeal joint spaces (arrows), thickening of the soft tissues of the hand (arrowhead), hypertrophy of the sesamoid bone of the thumb (black arrow).

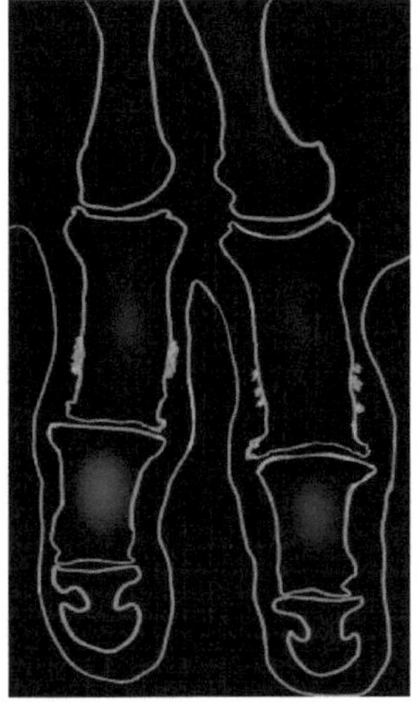

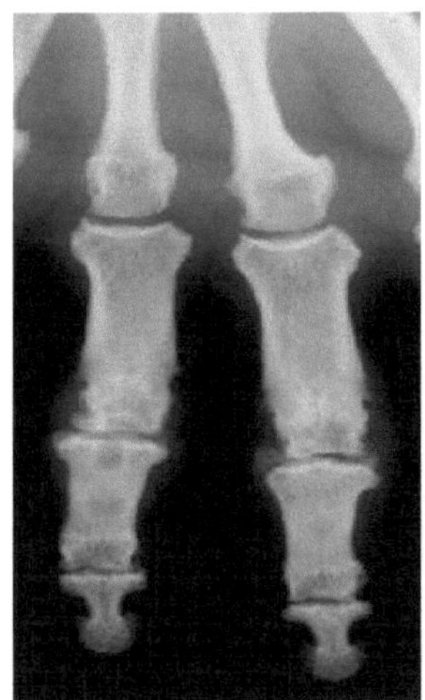

Fig. 7. Acromegaly. (a) Schematic diagram. (b) Finger X-ray, front. 1. Widening of joint spaces. 2. irregular muscle and tendon insertion zones. 3. Enlargement of phalangeal bases. 4 Osteophyte at base of 3rd phalanx. 5 Hypertrophy of phalangeal tuft with "anchor" osteophytes. 6. Thickening of soft tissue.

1.1.3.4.Spine

Radiological manifestations are most frequent in the dorsal and lumbar regions, with the following objectives (fig. 8):

- Accentuation of dorsal kyphosis and lumbar lordosis.
- Hypertrophy of the vertebral bodies.
- Enlargement of the anteroposterior diameter.
- Anteroposterior periosteal appositions.
- Anterolateral osteophytosis
- Posterior vertebral scalloping (accentuating the concavity of the posterior vertebral wall).

– Prevertebral ossifications.

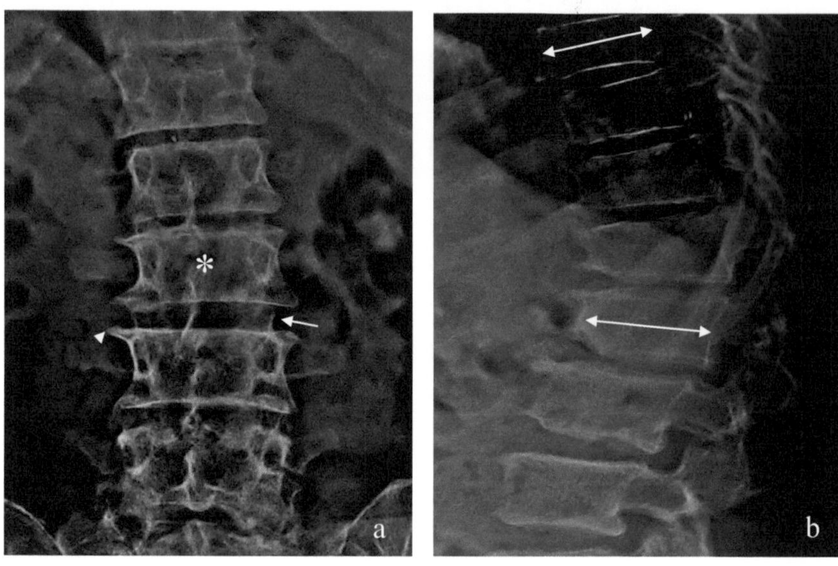

Fig. 8: Acromegaly. Radiographs of the spine: (a) Front lumbar; (b) Profile dorsolumbar. (a) Vertebral bodies appear enlarged, hypertrophied with no change in height (platyspondyly) (asterisk). Voluminous osteophytes (arrowhead). Enlargement of the intervertebral space (arrow). (b) Anteroposterior widening of the vertebral bodies of the lumbar spine (arrows, comparison with a normal overlying vertebral body).

1.1.3.5.Basin

In the pelvis, there is widening of the pubic symphysis, and changes to the coxofemoral and sacroiliac joints, with widening and pericapital osteophytosis (fig. 9).

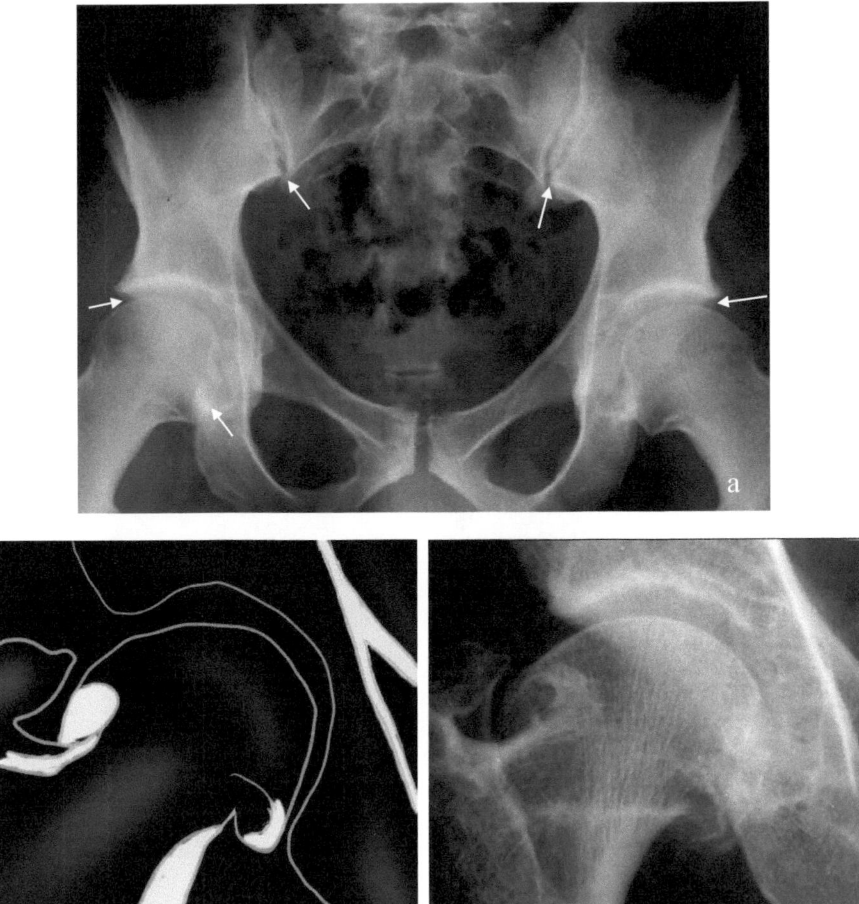

Fig. 9. Acromegaly. Standard radiographs. (a) Front pelvis. (b+ c) Diagram and enlargement of the coxofemoral joint. (a) Enlargement of pubic symphysis, coxofemoral joints and sacroiliac joints (arrow). (b) Enlargement of the hip joint with pericapital osteophytosis (arrowhead) [8].

1.1.3.6. Thorax

Hypertrophy of the costal cartilages is responsible for widening of the thoracic cage and opening of the sternal angle (fig. 10).

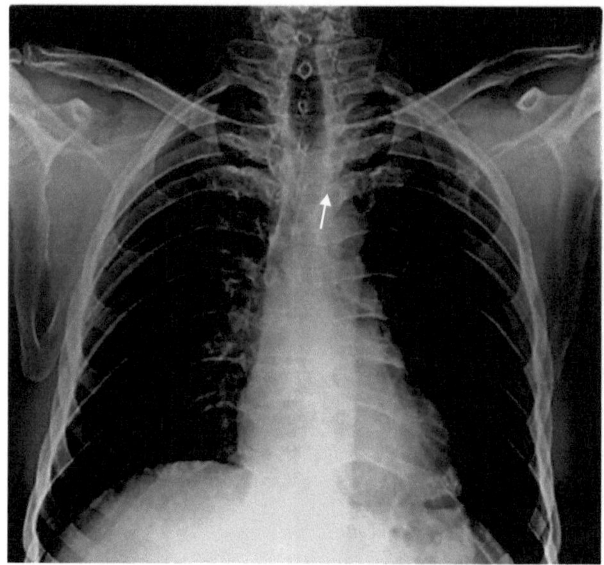

Fig. 10. Acromegaly. Standard chest X-ray. Opening of the sternal angle (arrow).

1.1.3.7.Other joints

All joints are subject to the changes described above (knee, hip, shoulder, ankle, etc.) (fig. 11). Thickening of tendon tissue (Achilles tendon), ductal syndromes and hyperostosis responsible for ossification at the entheses (as at the insertion of the superficial plantar fascia) can also be observed.

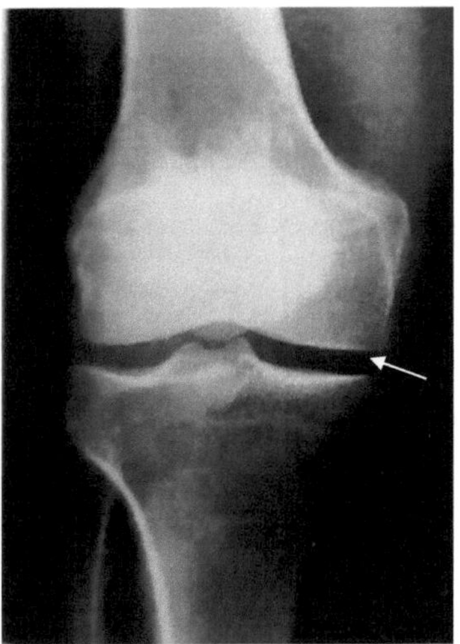
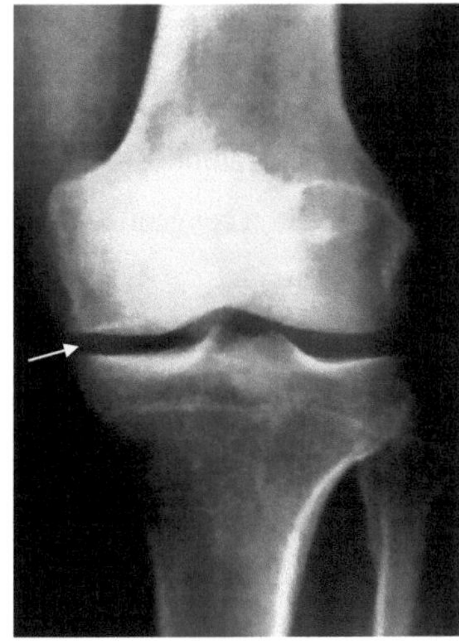

Fig. 11. Acromegaly. Standard radiographs of the front knees. Widening of the tibiofemoral interlines due to articular cartilage hypertrophy (arrows).

1.1.4. Differential diagnosis

The musculoskeletal manifestations of acromegaly are classically differentiated on imaging from pachydermoperiostosis (primary hypertrophic osteoarthropathy) [9].

Spinal manifestations may mimic spondyloarthropathy or Forestier's disease.

1.2. Hypopituitarism

Insufficient pituitary secretion can be caused by any lesion of the pituitary gland: trauma, surgery, tumors such as craniopharyngiomas, ischemia, etc. The main cause, however, is congenital. The main cause, however, is congenital.

1.2.1. Imaging

From birth, there is a delay in the appearance of ossification nuclei, which then become too small and irregular. This is often accompanied by osteopenia and delayed bone maturation. Complications can also be detected by the radiologist: osteopenia-related fractures [10], primary osteochondritis of the hip in children [11] and epiphysiolysis of the femoral head in adolescents [12].

In adults, osteoporosis can cause fractures [13].

1.3. Hyperprolactinemia

Excessive secretion of prolactin from the pituitary gland is most often due to iatrogenic medication.

Hyperprolactinemia accompanies hypopituitarism (removal of inhibition of prolactinemic secretion by hypothalamic dopamine). Hyperprolactinemia is accompanied by a significant decrease in bone mineral density, which appears to be related to hypogonadism [14].

2. Parathyroid

The four parathyroid glands are responsible for the secretion of parathyroid hormone (PTH). This hormone is responsible for maintaining calcium homeostasis via renal action through tubular reabsorption and vitamin D secretion, bone action through stimulation of resorption, and digestive action through increased calcium absorption by vitamin D.

2.1. Hyperparathyroidism

PTH hypersecretion by the parathyroid glands may be primitive, most often linked to a parathyroid adenoma, or secondary, linked to chronic hypocalcemia responsible for compensatory PTH hypersecretion by the parathyroids. Tertiary hyperparathyroidism also occurs when secondary hypersecretion persists despite normalization of the cause of hypocalcemia by autonomization of hypersecretion. Hyperparathyroidism is a frequent endocrinopathy whose incidence is increasing, and which mainly affects post-menopausal women (sex ratio equal to 2.5) [15, 16].

2.1.1. Clinic

Most hyperparathyroidism is asymptomatic, discovered incidentally during a laboratory work-up or cervical ultrasound [14].

Hypercalcemia may be symptomatic:

- Kidney lithiasis, gastrointestinal symptoms, pancreatitis,
- osteo-articular: mechanical pain, fractures, arthralgia, joint deformities,
- asthenia, neuropsychiatric disorders, cardiovascular disorders, hypertension, neuromuscular disorders.

2.1.2. Biology

Hypercalcemia is constant and PTH is generally elevated. Hypophosphatemia is often associated. Urinary calcium and phosphate excretion may also be increased.

2.1.3. Imaging

The main indication for imaging in hyperparathyroidism is the search for parathyroid adenoma by cervical ultrasound. CT and MRI are sometimes useful (fig. 11), as is methoxy-isobutyl-isonitrile (MIBI) scintigraphy for parathyroid adenoma in ectopic position [17].

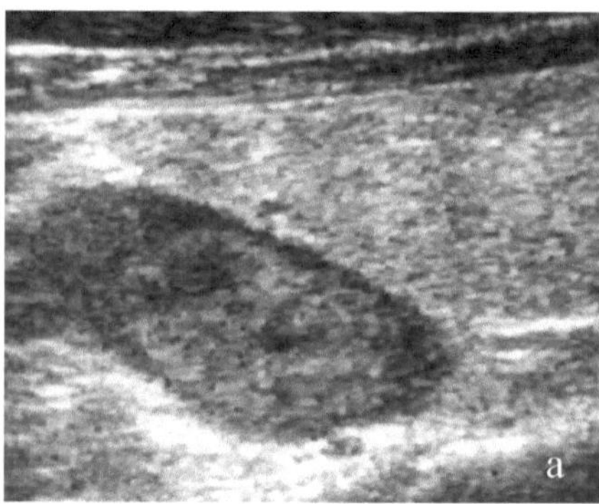

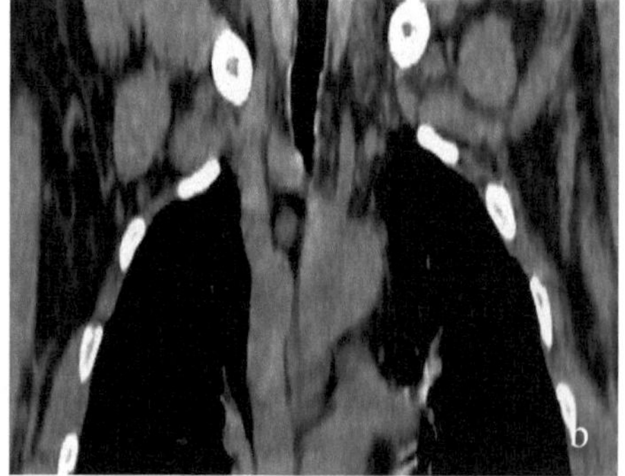

Fig. 11. parathyroid adenoma. (a) . Ultrasonography. Parathyroid mass, homogeneous hypoechoic, well limited. (b). Cervicothoracic CT scan. Ectopic localization of parathyroid adenoma (arrow).

The osteoarticular manifestations of hyperparathyroidism are accompanied by a wealth of radiological findings.

2.1.3.1.Bone resorption

It can be detected early in the hands. Bone resorption is found in multiple topographies: subperiosteal, intracortical, endosteal, trabecular, subchondral and at the entheses.

- **Subperiosteal resorption**

It is manifested by an irregularity of the outer edge of the bone cortex, which may take on a spiculated or "postage stamp" appearance. The topography of this resorption is suggestive: it often involves the phalangeal tassels (acro-osteolysis) and the radial edge of the phalanges, particularly the intermediate phalanges of the 2[e] and 3[e] radii (fig. 12).

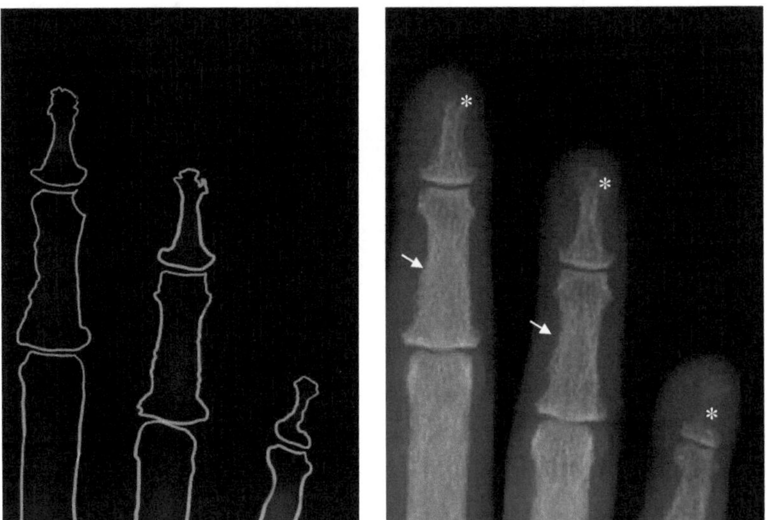

Fig. 12: Subperiosteal resorption (a) Diagram. (b) Finger X-ray, front view. Irregular resorption of the subperiosteal side of the cortex (nibbled appearance), predominantly on the radial edge of the 2nd phalanx (arrows). Resorption of phalangeal tufts (Acro-osteolysis) (asterisk).

Endo-cortical resorption

Endo-cortical resorption is manifested by a thinned cortex with a laminated appearance in relation to intacortical bone resorption (figs. 13, 14 and 15).

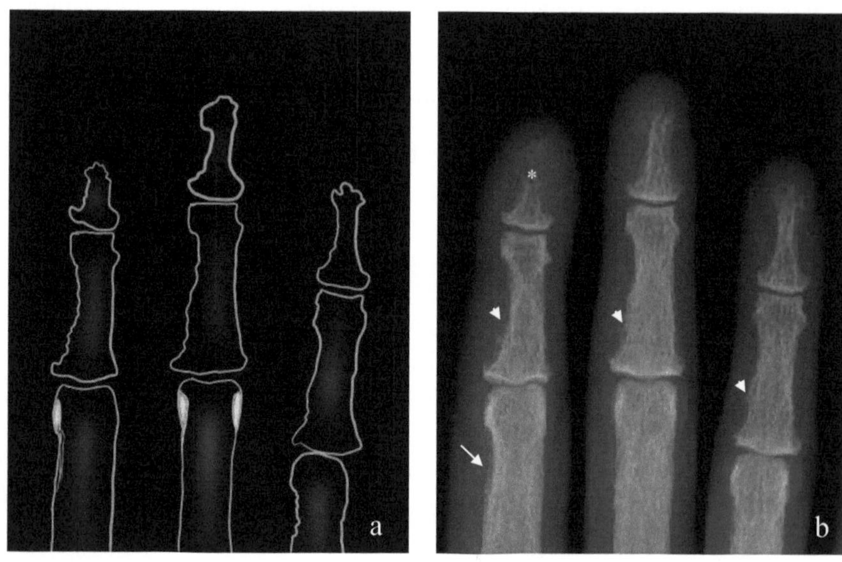

Fig. 13. Endo-cortical resorption. (a) Schematic diagram. (b) Facing radiograph of fingers. Clear vertical striae, with a laminated appearance of the cortex (arrow). There is associated subperiosteal resorption with irregular resorption of the subperiosteal side of the cortex, with a nibbled appearance, predominating on the radial edge of the 2nd phalanx of the 2nd and 3rd fingers (arrowhead). Resorption of phalangeal tassels (Acro-osteolysis) (asterisk).

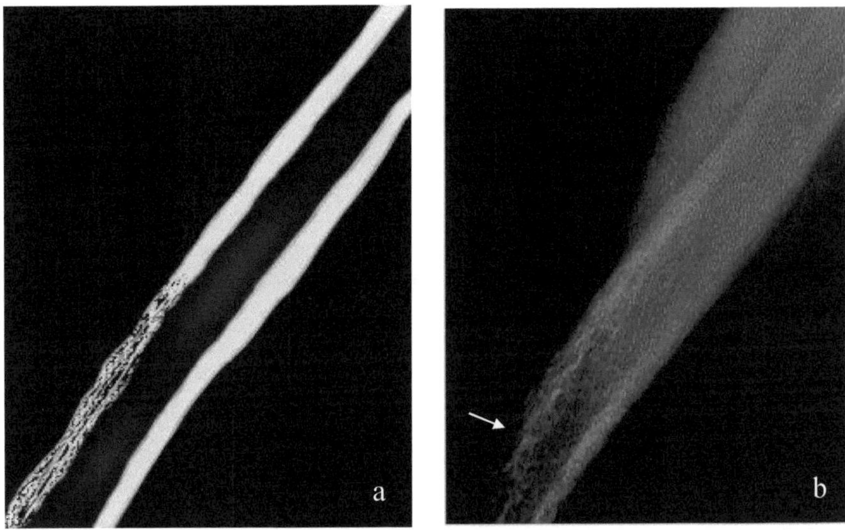

Fig. 14. Endo-cortical resorption. (a) Schematic diagram. (b) Radiograph of a long bone. Clear vertical striae, giving a laminated appearance to the cortex (arrow).

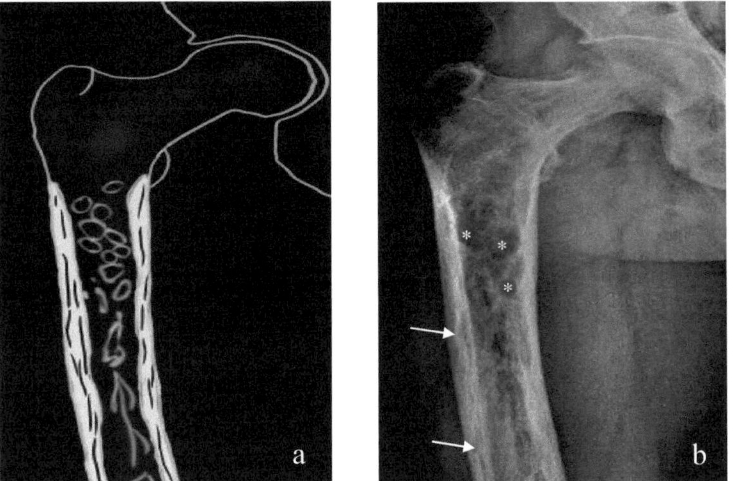

Fig. 15. Endo-cortical resorption. (a) Schematic diagram. (b) Radiograph of femur. Clear vertical striae, giving a laminated appearance to the cortex (arrow), associated with intramedullary osteolysis (asterisk).

• Trabecular resorption

This resorption is responsible for a "salt-and-pepper" appearance associated with a blurred appearance of the bone tables (fig. 16).

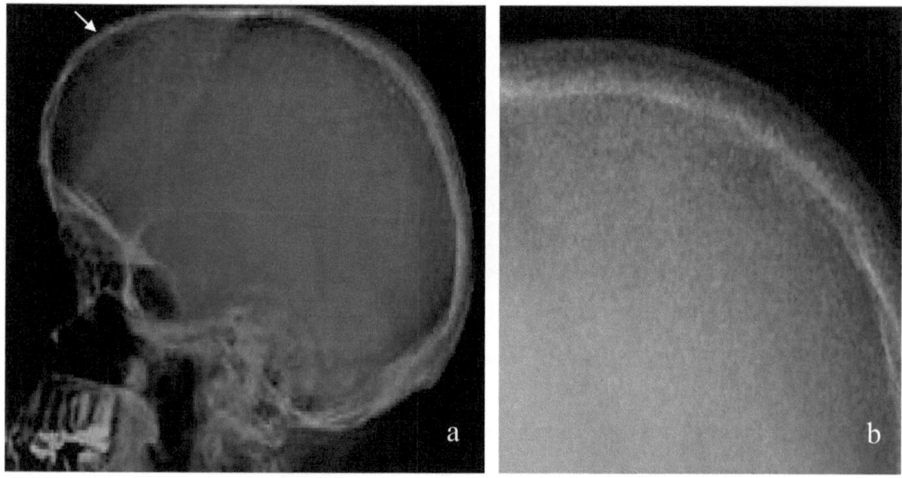

Fig. 16. Trabecular resorption. (a) Radiograph of the skull in profile. (b) Magnification. Granular, salt-and-pepper appearance of the bone structure. Thinning of the vault (arrow).

• Subchondral resorption

Subchondral resorption mainly affects the axial skeleton and girdles. It is characterized by irregular widening of the acromioclavicular interlines through resorption of the clavicular side, sacroiliac interlines and symphysis pubis [18] (figs. 17, 18 and 19). This resorption is manifested by extensive subchondral and juxtatendinous erosions, more or less associated with contact condensation (fig. 20).

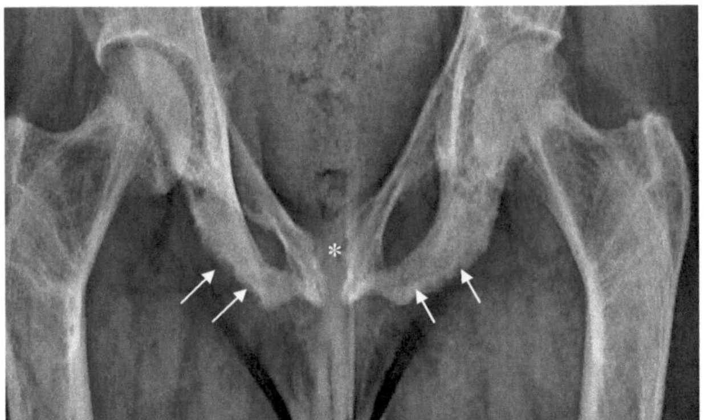

Fig. 17. Subchondral resorption. Radiograph of the pelvis. Irregular enlargement of the pubic symphysis (asterisk), subchondral erosions at the insertion of the entheses (arrows).

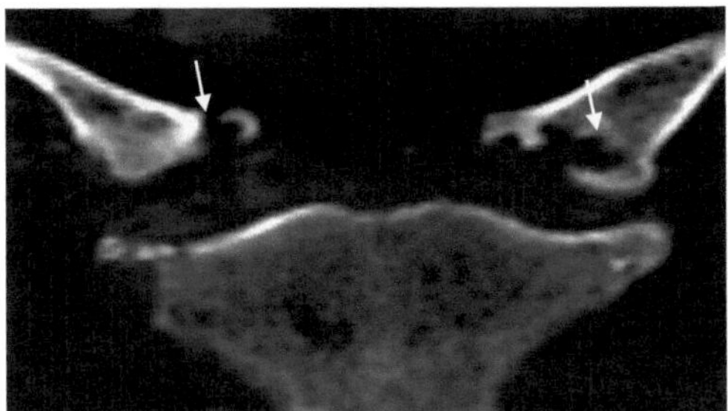

Fig. 18. Subchondral resorption. CT scan with coronal reconstruction centred on the clavicles. Clavicular subchondral geodes (arrows).

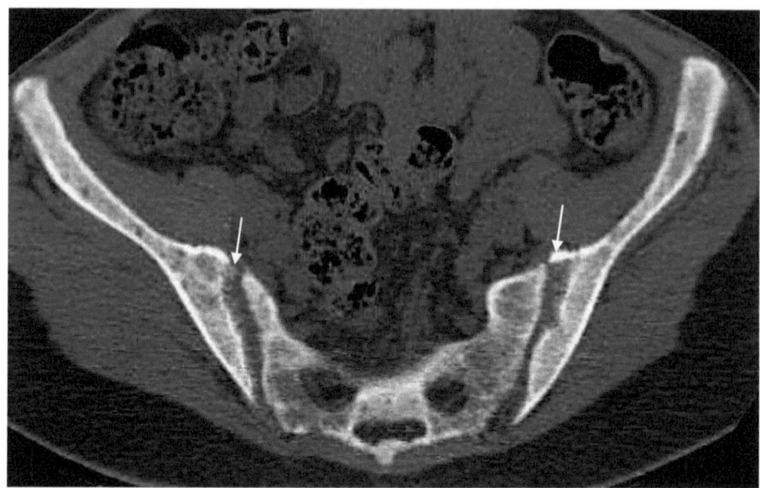

Fig. 19. Subchondral resorption. Bone window CT scan. Irregular enlargement of the sacroiliac joints (arrows).

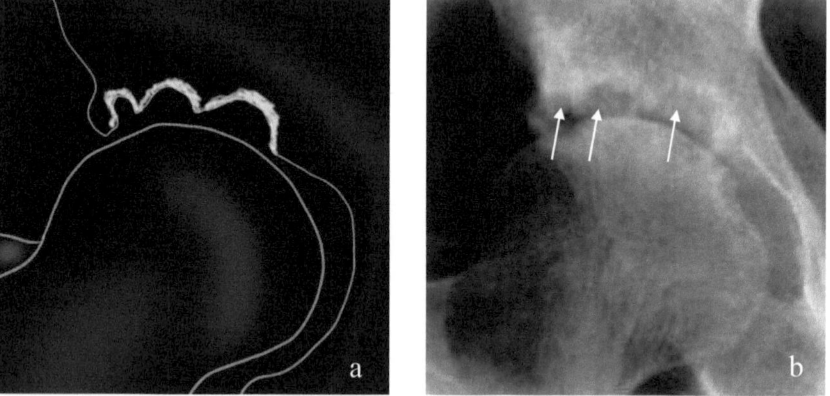

Fig. 20. Subchondral resorption. (a) Diagram. (b) Radiograph of the hip joint. Subchondral geodes surrounded by peripheral sclerosis (arrows).

2.1.3.2.Osteopenia

Osteoporosis is the rarefaction of the bone structure, often revealed by fracture complications (fig. 21).

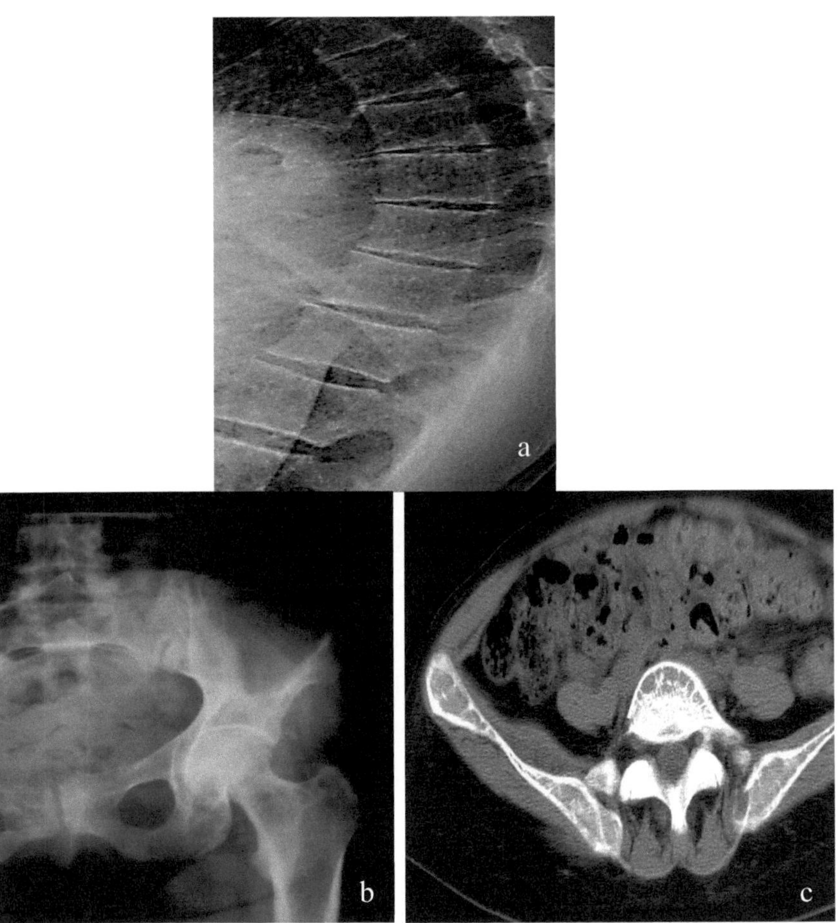

Fig. 21 Osteopenia (a). Radiograph of the spine in profile. (b) Front hip X-ray (c). CT scan of pelvis. Rarefaction of the bone structure, giving the appearance of empty vertebrae.

2.1.3.3.Brown tumors

These lesions are in fact pseudotumors formed by a more or less cystic hypervascularized fibrous tissue, containing numerous osteoclastic giant cells and often presenting hemosiderin deposits due to chronic intralesional microhemorrhages, responsible for the brown color of the lesion. They can be seen in around 3% of primary hyperparathyroidism cases [19, 20].

They mainly affect the limbs, such as the femurs and hands, but can also affect the mandible, pelvis, clavicles, ribs and spine. They are often asymptomatic, but sometimes manifest as swellings, fractures and bone pain.

On standard radiography, brown tumours present as lytic lesions, single or multiple, well-limited, without peripheral sclerosis, of cortical and eccentric topography, and may be accompanied by blown or even ruptured cortex [21] (figs. 22, 23). CT is indicated for exploration of areas that are difficult to analyze (fig. 24).

On MRI, the lesion presents as T1 hyposignal, tissue T2 hypersignal and strongly enhances after gadolinium injection [22, 23] (fig. 25). The T2 signal is sometimes heterogeneous, notably due to hemosiderin deposits in frank T2 hyposignal [24]. Necrotic remodeling may also be visible within these lesions, with a cystic, uni- or multilocular, or mixed, solidocystic appearance in T2 hypersignal, and their walls strongly enhanced after injection. Liquid-liquid levels may be visualized within cysts, mimicking an aneurysmal cyst [24].

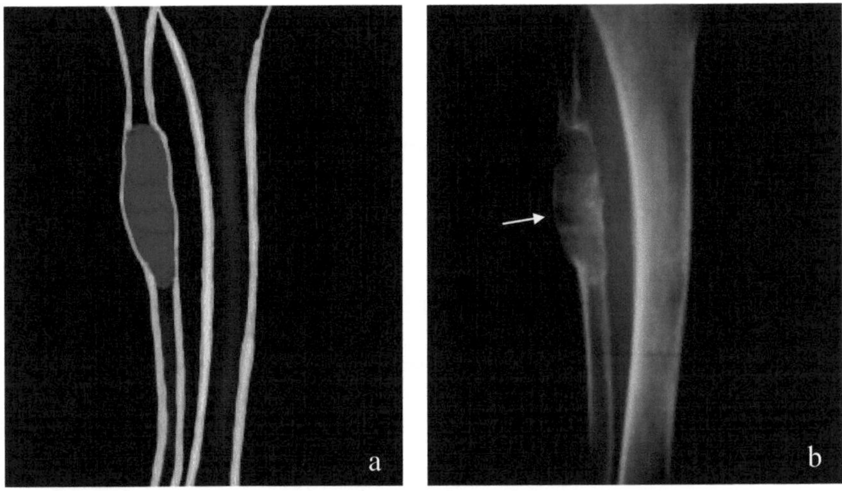

Fig. 22. Brown tumour (a) Diagram. (b) Front X-ray of the leg. Lytic lesion, located in the middle 1/3 of the fibula shaft, heterogeneous pattern, well limited, without peripheral sclerosis, blowing out the cortex, without rupture (arrow).

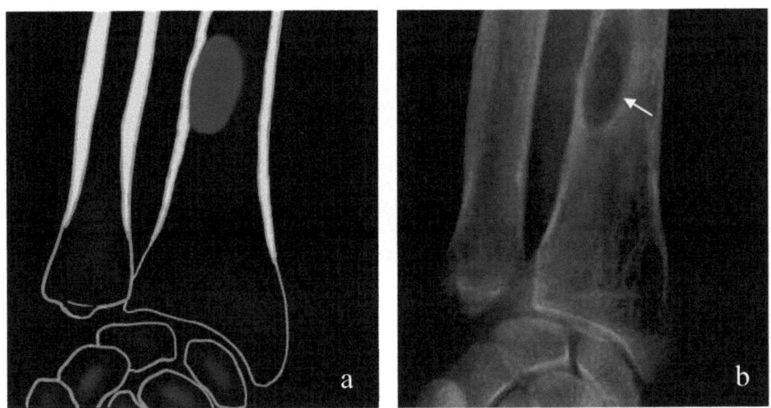

Fig. 23. Brown tumour (a) Schematic diagram. (b) Front X-ray of forearm. Osteolytic lesion, located in the lower 1/3 of the radial diaphysis, homogeneous, well limited, without peripheral sclerosis, cortical thinning, without rupture

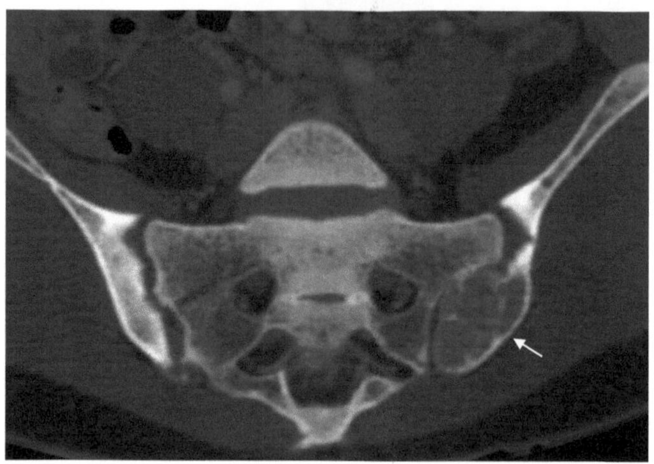

Fig. 24. Brown tumor. CT bone window. Left iliac lytic expansive process, containing septa, blowing cortical bone (arrow).

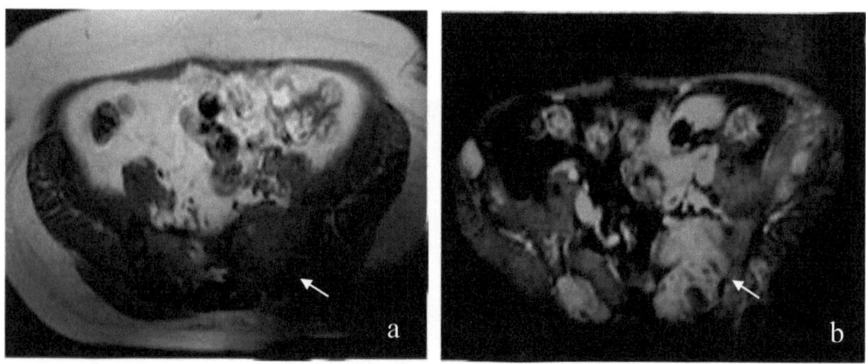

Fig. 25. Brown tumor. Brown tumour (a). MRI section of the hip, T1 sequence (b). MRI section of the hip, T1 sequence after injection of contrast medium. Mass of the sacral bone, in T1 hyposignal, enhancing after injection of gadolinium (arrows).

2.1.3.4. Osteosclerosis

Focal areas of osteosclerosis, mainly affecting the axial skeleton, may rarely be encountered in primary hyperparathyroidism (fig. 26).

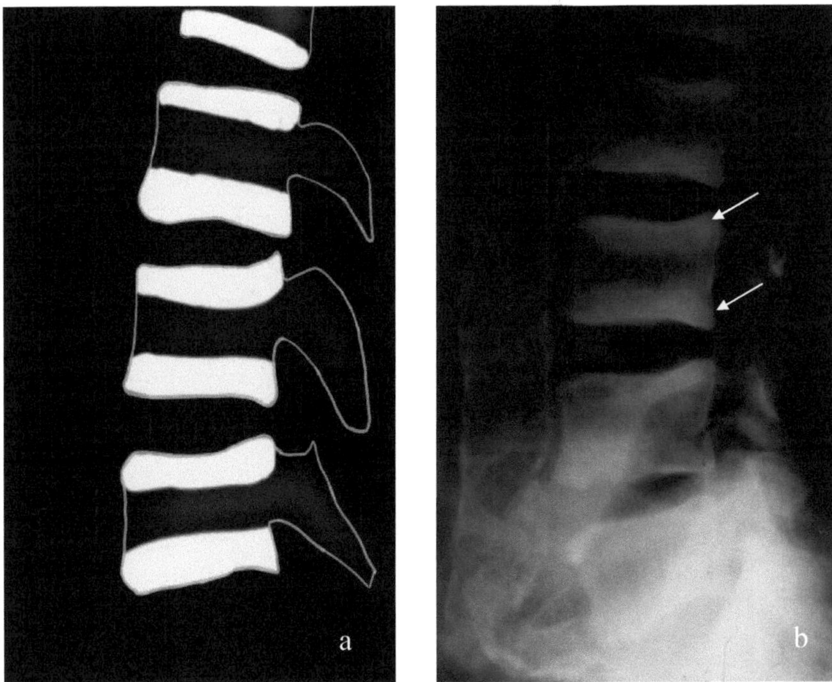

Fig. 26. osteosclerosis (a) diagram. (b) Radiograph of spine in profile. osteosclerosis in bands (arrows) "rugger jersey spine"; vertebrae "en maillot de rugby".

2.1.3.5.Heterotopic calcifications and tendinopathies

In the course of hyperparathyroidism, there is an increase in the frequency of disease with hydroxyapatite, calcium pyrophosphate and gout deposits [25]. These calcifications can occur in tendon structures and soft tissues (fig. 27).

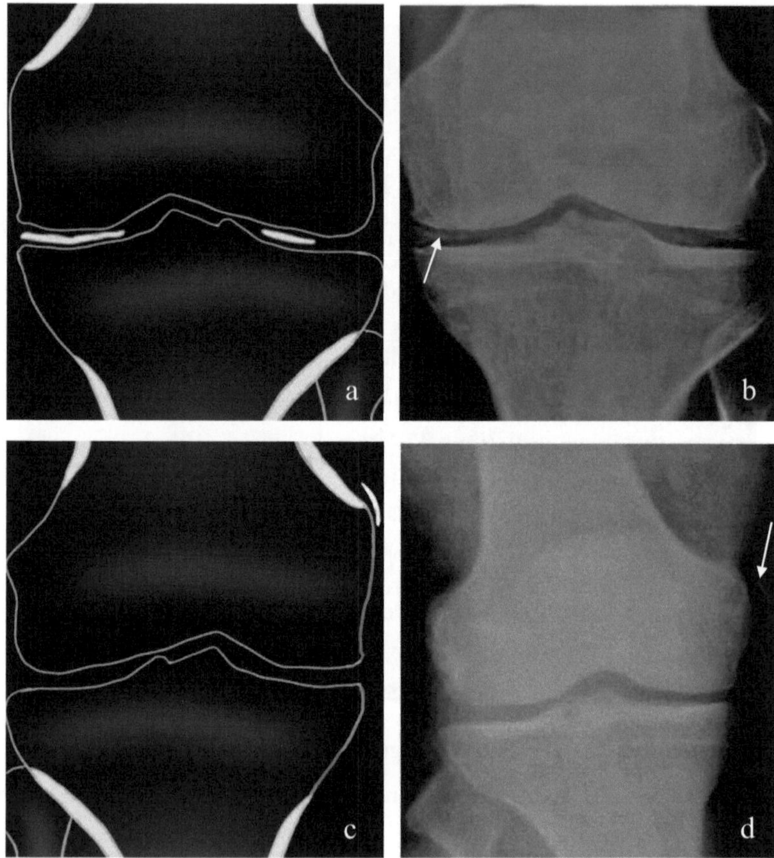

Fig. 27. Heterotopic calcifications and tendinopathies. (a) Diagram. (b) Front X-ray of knee. Joint calcifications caused by calcium pyrophosphate crystal deposition (arrow). (c) Diagram. (d) Calcification of the LLI (arrow).

2.1.4. Complications

In hyperparathyroidism, bone complications often include pathological fractures and bone deformities, such as thoracic deformity (fig. 28).

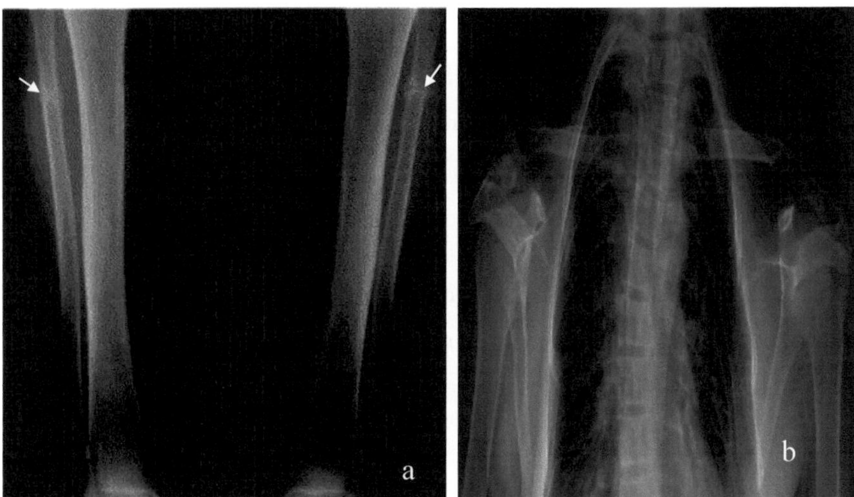

Fig. 28. Complications. (a) Front X-ray of both legs. Fracture line at fibula level (arrows). (b) Front thoracic X-ray. Thoracic deformity.

2.2. Hypoparathyroidism

Hypoparathyroidism can be acquired, idiopathic, especially in women, or iatrogenic, secondary to surgical removal or destruction by irradiation.

2.2.1. Clinic

Profound hypocalcemia can lead to muscle cramps, neurological disorders such as paresthesias and convulsions, but also mental deterioration and long-term disorders of the dentition and phanera [26, 27].

2.2.2. Biology

Hypoparathyroidism is generally accompanied by a decrease in plasma PTH, hypocalcemia, hyperphosphatemia and a decrease in vitamin D.

2.2.3. Imaging

There is a significant overall increase in bone density in the form of focused osteocondensation in dense metaphyseal bands, densification of the iliac crests and thickening of the cranial vault, as well as spinal hyperostosis and ossifying enthesopathies [28-30] (fig. 29). Defects of dentition can be observed in the facial region [31].

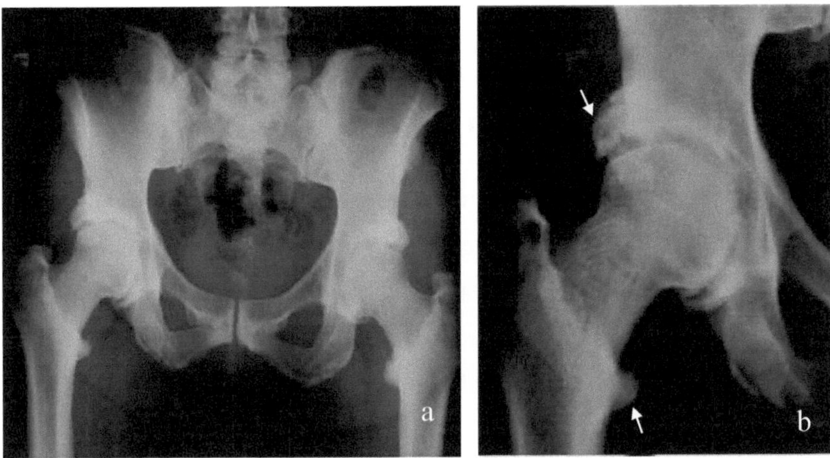

Fig. 29. Hypoparathyroidism. (a) Radiograph of pelvis. (b) Radiograph of hip. Overall increase in bone mineral density, densification of iliac crests and ossifying enthesopathies (arrows) [6].

3. Thyroid

Thyroid hormones (T3, T4) are activators of basic metabolism. In children, they play a key role in the growth and maturation of bone tissue.

3.1. Hyperthyroidism

Excess thyroid hormone leads to accelerated bone remodeling and excessive catabolism, resulting in bone demineralization. Hyperthyroidism is of primary etiology, of thyroid origin such as Graves' disease, toxic adenoma, multinodular goiter, etc... More rarely, it is secondary to TSH hypersecretion by the pituitary gland, secondary to a pituitary adenoma.

3.1.1. Clinic

Clinical signs are those of a global increase in basal metabolism: hypersudation, tachycardia, tremors, nervousness, weight loss, diarrhea, etc. Pathological fractures are often found, due to bone resorption [32, 33]. In Graves' disease, the symptomatology is that of Diamond's triad, which includes pretibial myxedema, exophthalmos and acropathy (edema of the fingers and toes and digital hippocratism). In children, hyperthyroidism leads to accelerated bone maturation and premature fusion of growth plate.

3.1.2. Biology

The diagnosis is made biologically, by measuring TSH, which is decreased, and free T4, which is increased. Hypercalciuria and even hypercalcemia may be present.

3.1.3. Imaging

3.1.3.1.Bone thinning

The severity of osteoporosis can be assessed by bone densitometry and is correlated with the extent of thyroid hormone hypersecretion [33].

Bone rarefaction mainly affects the cortical bone, giving the striated, laminated appearance of the cortical bone, visible especially in the extremities (fig. 30). The cranial vault may also be affected, with increased visibility of the vascular grooves, giving the appearance of pseudomyeloma (fig. 31) [4].

Pathological fracture is the main complication of osteoporosis, often involving the femoral neck and spine.

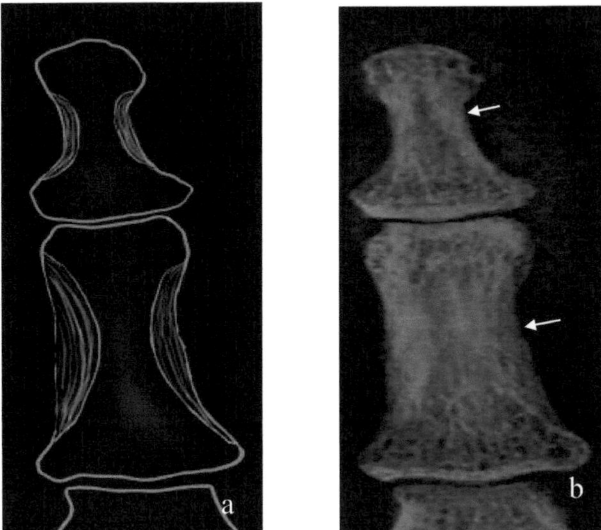

Fig. 30. Bone rarefaction (a) Diagram. (b) Radiograph of fingers. Bone rarefaction predominantly in the cortical bone, which takes on a thinned, laminated appearance (arrows) [6].

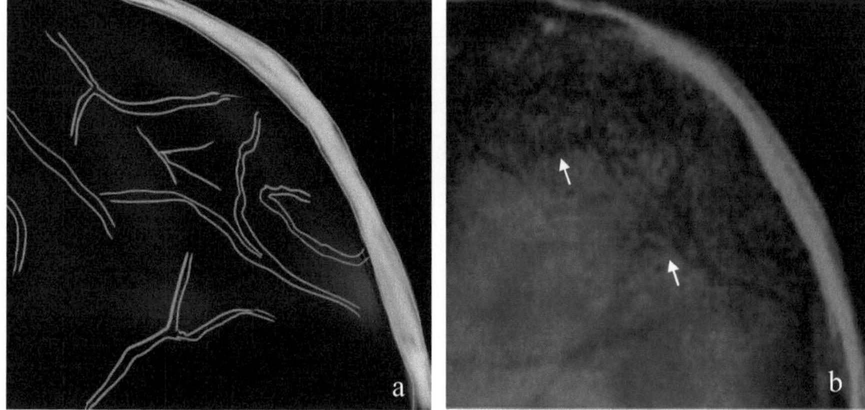

Fig. 31. Bone rarefaction (a) Diagram. (b) Skull radiograph in profile. Bone rarefaction responsible for improved visibility of vascular grooves, which can lead to a pseudomyeloma appearance (arrows) [6].

3.1.3.2.Thyroid acropachy

Irregular, "sinuous" and asymmetrical periosteal reactions on the diaphyses of the metacarpals, phalanges or metatarsals [34] (fig. 32). This reaction is predominant on the radial side of the 1st and 2nd metacarpals, and on the ulnar side of the 5th metacarpal. An increase in the diaphyseal diameter of the metacarpals, phalanges and metatarsals can also be observed, due to cortical thickening (fig. 33).

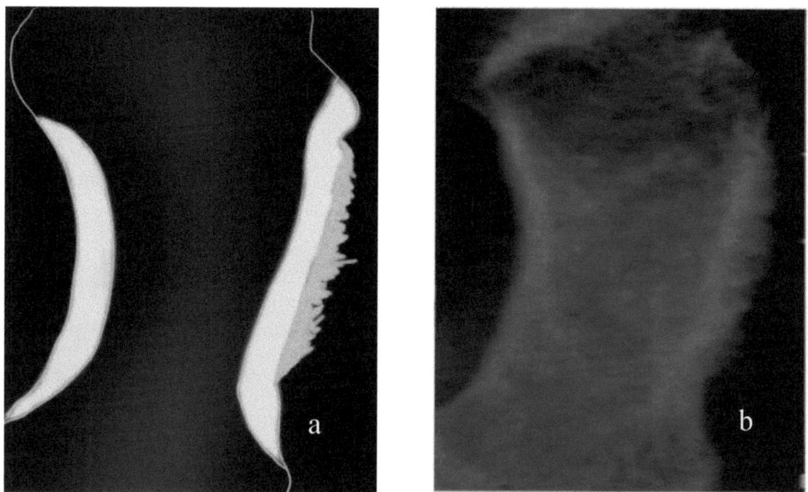

Fig. 32. Thyroid acropachy. (a) Schematic diagram. (b) Details of a hand X-ray. Asymmetric, irregular, sinuous periosteal reaction located on the metacarpal diaphyses (arrow) [6].

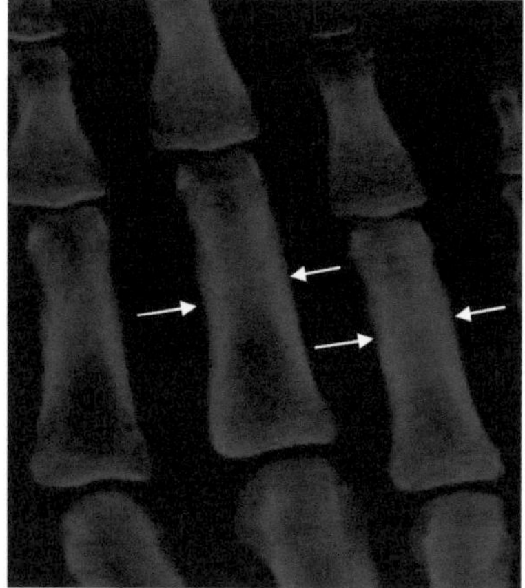

Fig. 33. Thyroid acropachy. Details of a hand X-ray. Increase in diaphyseal diameter of phalanges (arrow).

3.2. Hypothyroidism

Hypothyroidism is the insufficiency of thyroid hormones, which is responsible for a drop in basal metabolism. It is generally congenital in children. In adults, hypothyroidism is often of primary origin (infectious, iatrogenic, tumoral, etc.).

3.2.1. Clinic

In newborns, hypothyroidism manifests as jaundice, macroglossia, hypotonia and epiphyseal dysgenesis. In untreated children, the disease presents with dwarfism and mental retardation [35, 36]. In adults, the symptoms of hypometabolism include depression, constipation, bradycardia, weight gain, psychomotor retardation, mucosal infiltration and skin dryness.

3.2.2. Biology

In hypothyroidism, there is an increase in serum TSH and a drop in serum free T4.

3.2.3. Imaging

From birth, a delay in the appearance and development of epiphyseal nuclei can be observed [24] (fig. 34). The morphology of the epiphyses is also abnormal, with an irregular, fragmented appearance (fig. 34). In the skull, delayed growth and bone maturation are manifested by the presence of Wormian bones and delayed closure of the sutures (brachycephaly due to delayed closure of the spheno-occipital synchondrosis), and delayed appearance of the para-nasal sinuses and mastoids. As regards the axial skeleton, there is hypoplasia of the anterosuperior angle of the vertebral bodies of the dorsolumbar hinge, giving a "rostrum" appearance responsible for kyphosis. In adults, non-specific osteocondensations, sometimes complicated by fractures, and soft-tissue calcifications are observed [37, 38]. The main symptomatic lesions are carpal tunnel syndrome and tenosynovitis.

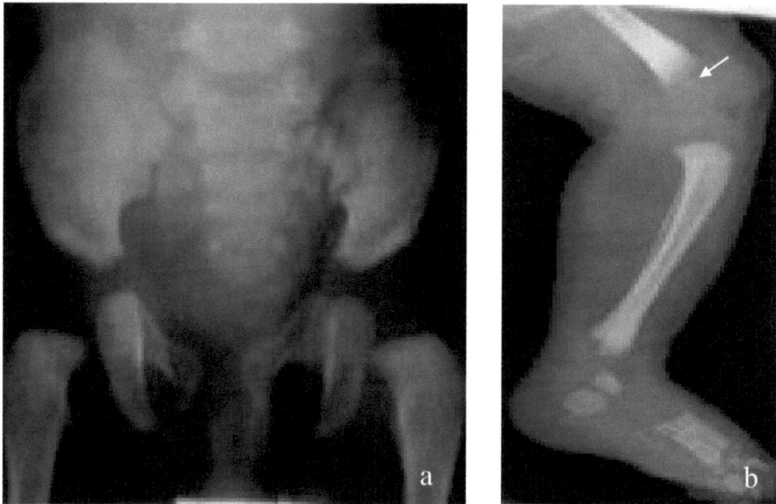

Fig. 34. Congenital hypothyroidism. (a) Front radiograph of the pelvis. Delayed appearance of epiphyseal nuclei in a full-term newborn. (b). Radiograph of the left leg in profile. Epiphyseal dysgenesis in a term newborn, irregular epiphysis (arrow) [6].

4. Adrenals

The adrenal glands are made up of two parts: the medullary adrenal gland, which secretes catecholamines, and the adrenal cortex, which secretes corticosteroids, primarily cortisol. Cortisol is a hormone that stimulates catabolism, particularly of bone.

4.1. Hypercorticism

Hypercorticism is the excess of glucocorticoid hormones, responsible for increased bone catabolism through activation of osteoclasts and inhibition of osteoblastic activity.

Hypercorticism can be endogenous, due to excess cortisol secretion caused by adrenal hyperplasia or pituitary adenoma. It can also be of iatrogenic origin, secondary to long-term treatment with steroidal anti-inflammatory drugs.

4.1.1. Clinic

Fasciotruncal obesity, diabetes, high blood pressure, nervousness, muscle weakness due to myopathy and amyotrophy, stretch marks on the skin and gonadal disorders are generally observed.

In children, osteoporosis is common, associated with delayed bone maturation [39].

4.1.2. Biology

Diagnosis is based on a 24-hour urine free cortisol (UFC) assay. A dexamethasone braking test may also be used to confirm the diagnosis. An ACTH assay may also be useful.

4.1.3. Imaging

4.1.3.1.Osteoporosis

Osteoporosis is generally visible in areas where trabecular bone predominates, such as the upper extremities of the femur and spine (fig. 35). Bone mineral density is reduced, with an increased risk of fracture, which in 70% of cases occurs in the lumbar spine [40, 41]. Rib fractures are also frequent [42].

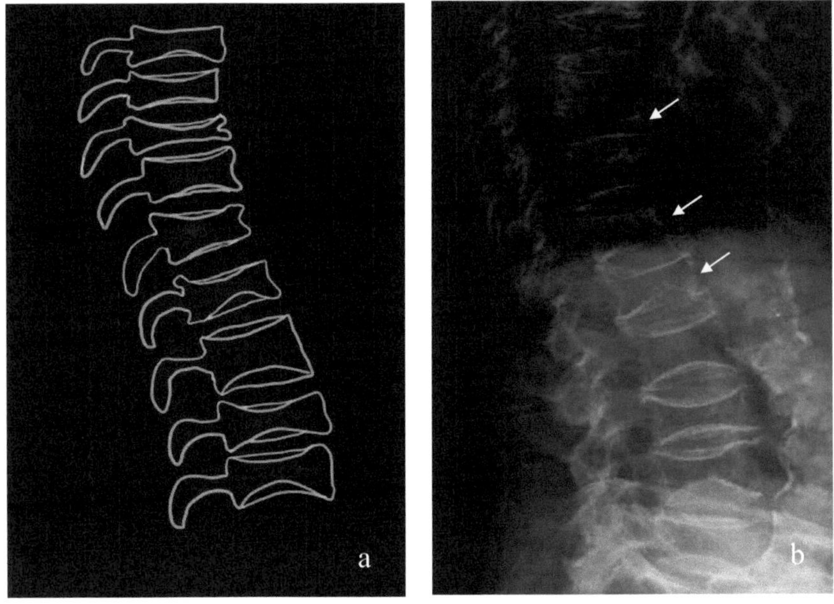

Fig. 35. Osteoporosis (a) Diagram. (b) Profile X-ray of lumbar spine. Osteoporosis giving the appearance of a vertebral void, complicated by stepped vertebral compression (arrows).

4.1.3.2. Aseptic osteonecrosis

Aseptic osteonecrosis is mainly seen in iatrogenic hypercorticism [43, 44]. They frequently involve the femoral heads and condyles, but also the humeral heads.

Clinically, aseptic osteonecrosis may be asymptomatic, and its characteristics are non-specific. However, their widespread, bilateral and multifocal nature may be suggestive.

On standard radiographs, the femoral head has a normal appearance at first, which does not rule out a positive diagnosis of aseptic osteonecrosis. Radiological changes are grouped into four Ficat stages:

- Stage 1: normal radiological appearance (fig. 36).
- Stage 2: segmental, heterogeneous demineralization of the femoral head "in quarters", with peripheral condensation. Contours of the femoral head are preserved. The hip joint and acetabulum are normal (Fig. 37).
- Stage 3: subsidence with loss of cephalic sphericity; ovalization or localized flattening of the femoral head; unhooking of the cephalic rim; appearance of linear subchondral clearness with eggshell pattern; more or less extensive oval or triangular hyperclearness, limited at its lower part by an upwardly concave band of osteosclerosis (fig. 38). The coxofemoral joint and acetabulum are normal.
- Stage 4: flattening of femoral head; dissection of necrotic bone (fig. 39).

In the terminal stage, joint pinching is observed, followed by coxarthrosis (Steinberg stages 5 and 6).

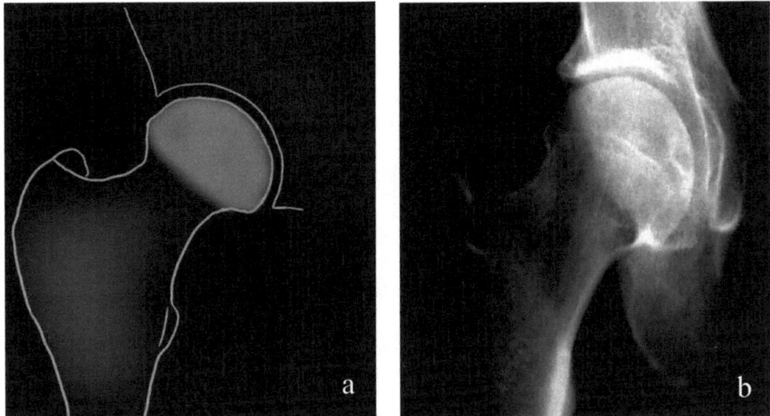

Fig. 36. Aseptic osteonecrosis. Ficat stage 1. (a) Schematic diagram. (b) Radiograph of the hip. Normal radiological appearance.

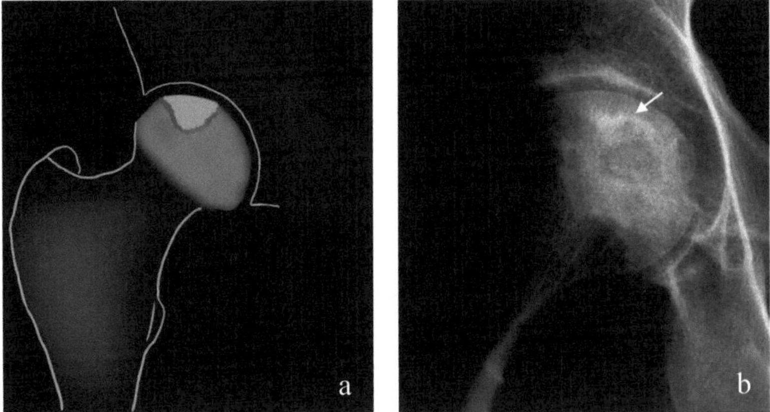

Fig. 37. Aseptic osteonecrosis. Ficat stage 2. (a) Schematic diagram. (b) Radiograph of the hip. Segmental, heterogeneous demineralization of the femoral head with peripheral condensation (arrow).

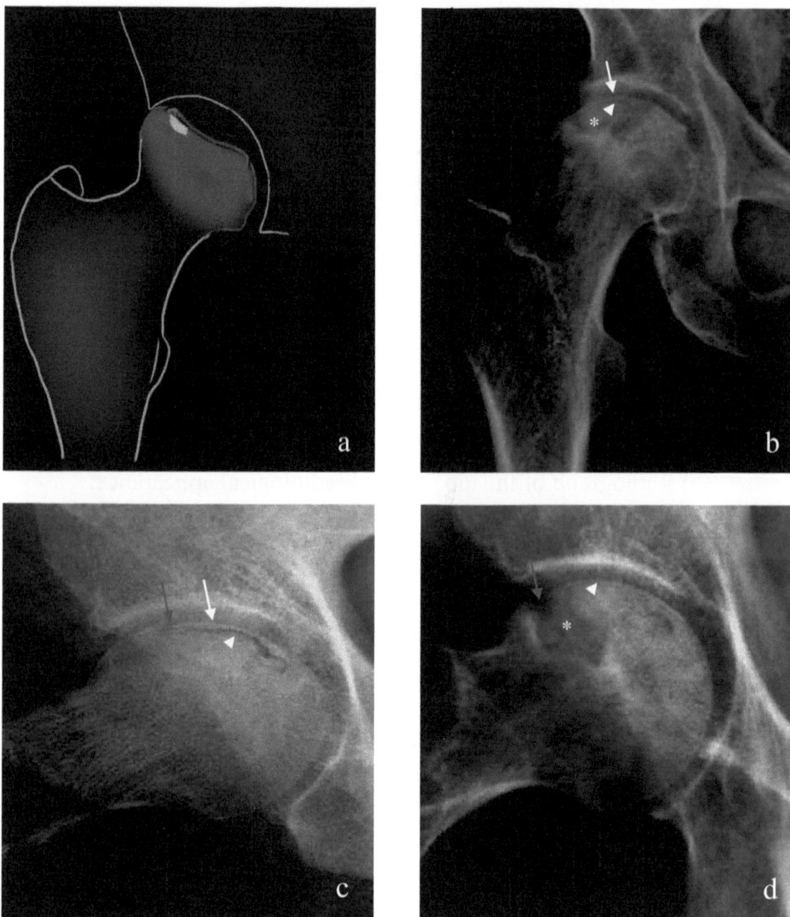

Fig. 38. Aseptic osteonecrosis. Ficat stage 3. (a) Schematic diagram. (b) Radiograph of the hip. (c+d) Enlargement. Localized flattening of the femoral head (white arrow). Oval or triangular hyperclarity, more or less extensive, limited in its lower part by an upwardly concave band of osteosclerosis (asterisk). Detachment of the cephalic rim (red arrow). Appearance of subchondral linear clarity with eggshell pattern (arrowhead).

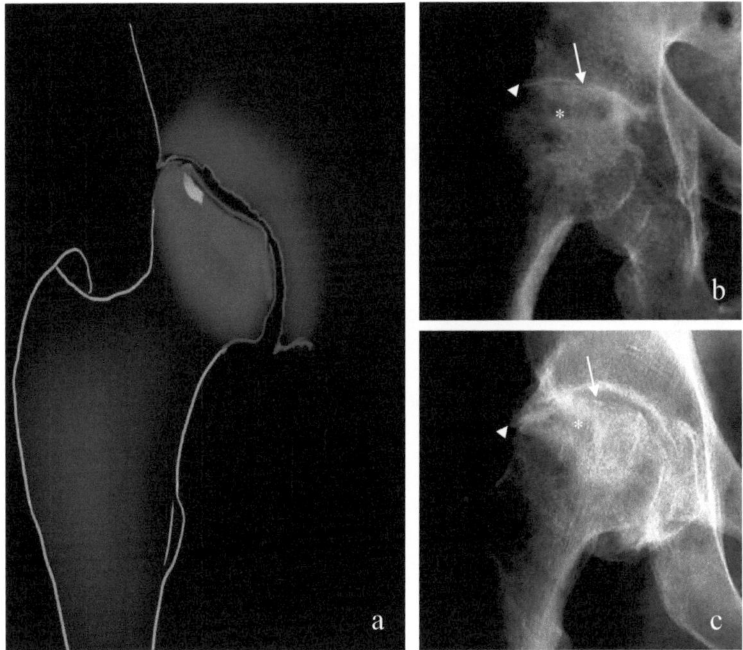

Fig. 39. Aseptic osteonecrosis. Ficat stage 4. (a) Schematic diagram. (b+c) Radiograph of the hip. Flattening of the femoral head (arrow), dissection of necrotic and heterogeneous bone (asterisk). Joint pinching and osteophytes (arrowhead).

On MRI, osteonecrosis appears as a geographically mapped zone of necrosis of variable signal, T1 hypersignal in the early stage, delimited by a border of T1 hyposignal and T2 hypersignal then T2 hyposignal once calcified (fig. 40).

This border may present as a double line, one in T2 hyposignal and the other in T2 hypersignal, best seen when fat signal is suppressed [45, 46]. The area of necrosis does not enhance after contrast injection. The lesion may be associated with T2 hypersignal peripheral bone edema and intra-articular effusion, especially if epiphyseal in location.

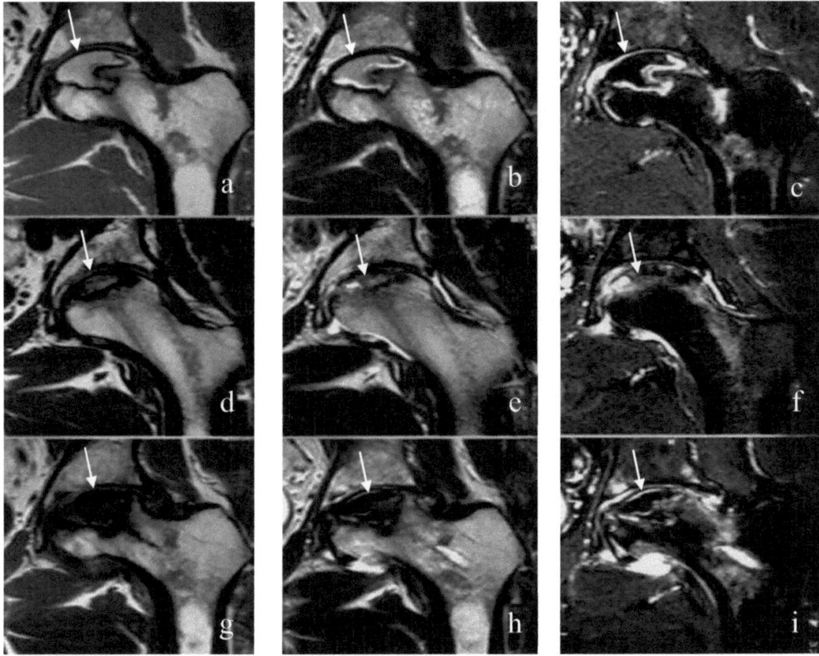

Fig. 40. Aseptic osteonecrosis. MRI: (a+d+g) T1-weighted sequence; (b+e+h) T2-weighted sequence; (c+f+i) T2-weighted Fat Sat sequence. Three types of sequestrum signal according to Mitchell: (a+b+c) Fat signal, T1, T2 hypersignal and T2 Fat Sat hyposignal; (d+e+f) Fluid signal, T1 hyposignal, T2 hypersignal and T2 Fat Sat hyposignal; (g+h+i) Fibrous signal, T1, T2 hyposignal and T2 Fat Sat hyposignal (arrows).

4.1.3.3.Epidural lipomatosis

Epidural lipomatosis corresponds to the accumulation of adipose tissue within the epidural space, generally at lumbar level, but may also affect other floors in cases of hypercorticism [47, 48] (fig. 41). It is rarely symptomatic, due to narrowing of the spinal canal and compression of the spinal roots. On MRI, lipomatosis is hypersignal T1, T2 and hyposignal T2 Fat Sat [49, 50].

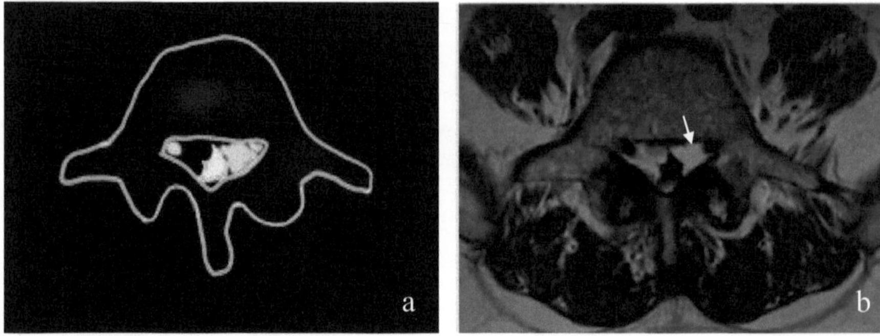

Fig. 41. Epidural lipomatosis secondary to Cushing's disease. (a) Schematic diagram. (b) MRI of the lumbar spine in T1 sequence in the transverse plane. Epidural fatty tissue thickening in T1 hypersignal, responsible for a reduction in the caliber of the dural sac (arrow) [6].

5. Pancreas

5.1. Diabetes

Diabetes mellitus is defined as high blood sugar levels, due to a deficiency of the pancreatic hormone insulin, which corresponds to type 1 diabetes, or peripheral resistance to this hormone, which corresponds to type 2 diabetes. There are many complications associated with diabetes, including osteoarticular, cardiac, renal and ocular complications.

5.1.1. Diabetic foot

Diabetic foot is a frequent and serious complication of diabetes. It affects around 15% of patients, and in 10% of cases leads to limb amputation [51, 52].

The pathophysiology of this complication is multifactorial. Chronic hyperglycemia leads to sensory neuropathy, which is responsible for the occurrence of painless microtrauma wounds. It is also responsible for microangiopathy, which leads to poor wound healing. Over time, the neuropathy becomes motoric, and is responsible for foot deformity, increasing the risk of ulceration by modifying areas of cutaneous hyperpressure (fig. 42). Later, bone resorption sets in, with fragmentation and joint dislocation, leading to Charcot's foot. This pathophysiological phenomenon is aggravated by the increased susceptibility of diabetic patients to infections [53] (fig. 43).

The diabetic foot is a combination of nerve osteoarthropathy and infectious osteoarthropathy.

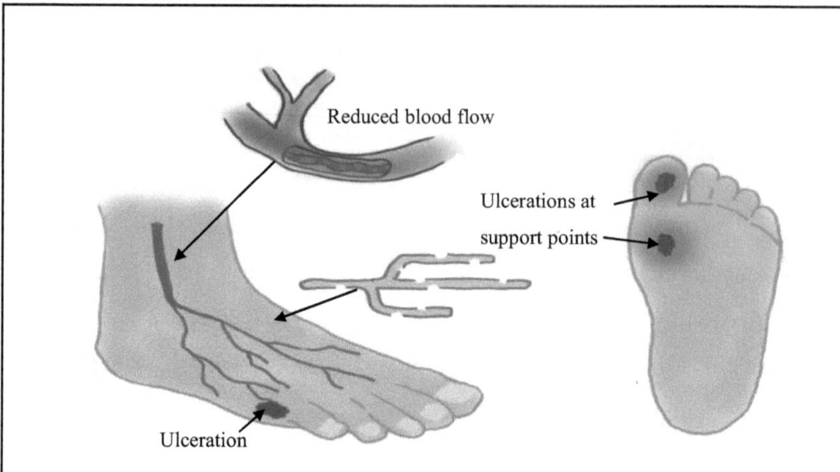

Fig. 42. Diagram of the pathophysiology of diabetic foot ulceration.

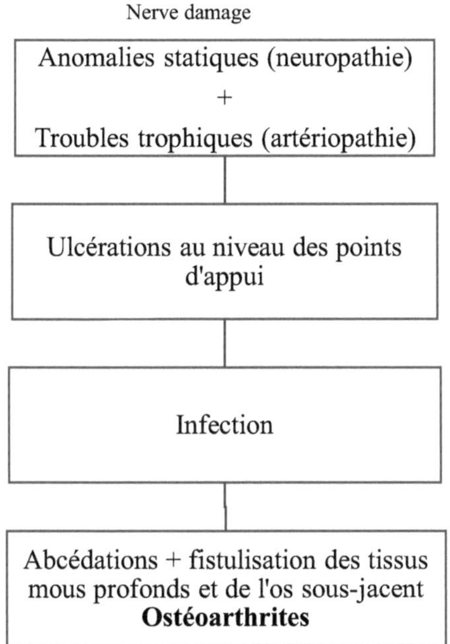

Fig. 43. Pathophysiology of the diabetic foot

5.1.1.1.Nervous osteoarthropathy

The preferred site is the tarsal bones (60%). There are two clinical forms: atrophic (osteoporosis, bone resorption, dislocation, disintegration within a few weeks) and hypertrophic (osteophytes, sclerosis, eburnation, fragmentation, dislocation). Static disorders are the main lesions encountered in diabetic neuroarthriopathies, such as collapse, plantar dislocation, metatarsal head dislocation, claw toe, metatarsophalangeal subluxation and bone destruction.

- **Imaging**

In the case of diabetic foot, bone manifestations warrant comparative standard radiographs of both feet, front and side. The indications for standard radiographs are :

- In all patients with diabetic neuroarthropathy.

- Any patient with a plantar ulcer.

- To assess the extent of lesions.

- For ongoing monitoring.

In the early stages of nerve osteoarthropathy, standard X-rays may be normal or may show mediacalcosis, which corresponds to vascular calcifications in a rail underlining the vascular pathway (fig. 44). Progressively, signs of subchondral bone rarefaction can be seen, usually at the heads of the metatarsals (fig. 44). Subsequently, X-rays reveal arthropathy with the appearance of osteoarthritis. The diagnosis of nerve osteoarthropathy is made when the patient is diabetic, the disease progresses rapidly and, above all, the lesions are located in a specific area [53]. The predictive location for nerve osteoarthropathy is the medial column of the foot, in contact with the navicular bone and medial cuneiform [54]. Joint pinching with subchondral geodes, subchondral osteosclerosis and osteophytes are evident. The progression is towards joint dislocation and destruction (fig. 45). In the late stage, arthropathy progresses to ankylosis of the foot, with the presence of intra-articular foreign bodies, culminating in Charcot's flat, cuboid foot [53] (fig. 46).

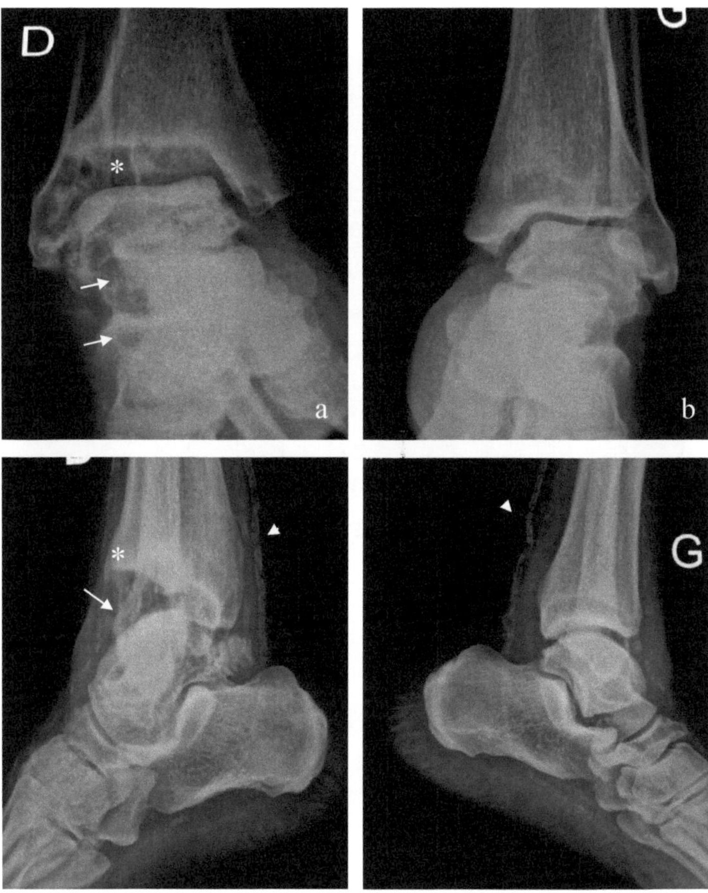

Fig. 44. Nerve osteoarthropathy. (a+b) Standard frontal radiographs of bilateral ankles, comparative. (c+d) Standard profile radiographs of bilateral ankles. Right tibial subchondral osteolysis (asterisk), associated with talus subchondral geodes (arrow). Mediacalcosis, vascular rail calcifications highlighting the vascular pathway (arrowhead).

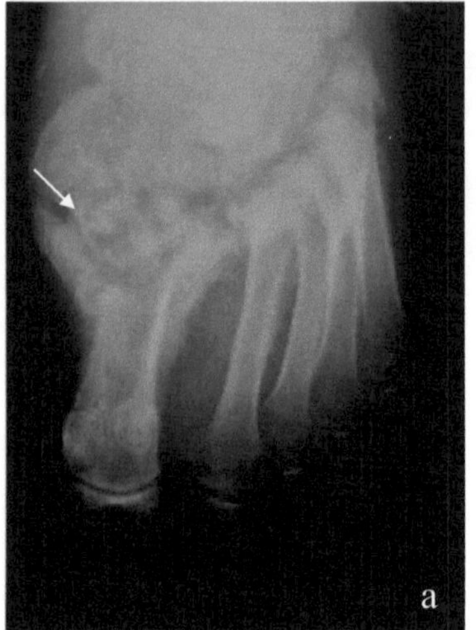

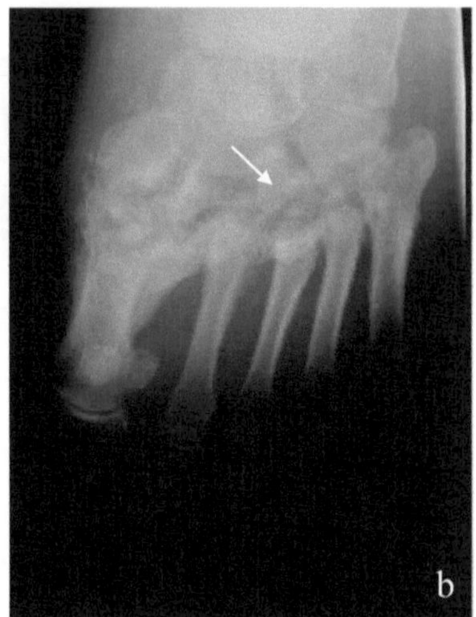

Fig. 45. Nerve osteoarthropathy. (a+b) Standard radiographs of the front forefoot. (a) Dislocation and joint destruction, associated with intra-articular foreign bodies (arrow). (b) Joint ankylosis (arrow).

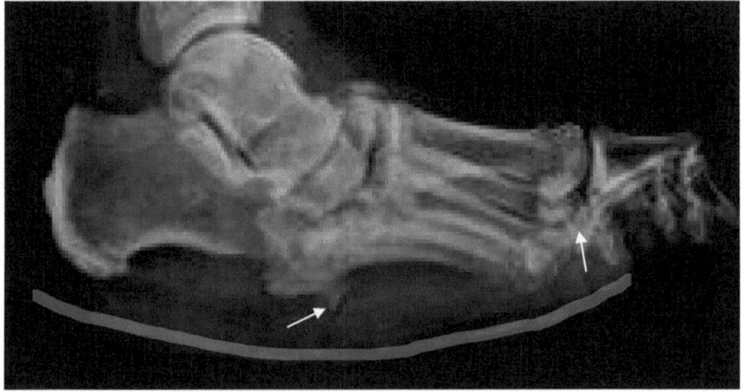

Fig. 46. Charcot foot. Standard radiograph of the foot in profile. Osteophytes (arrows). Foot deformity.

The resorptive form may be observed [51]. Preferentially located in the metatarsophalangeal joints, it presents as progressive osteolysis with sharp, well-defined edges, giving a tapered shape to the metatarsal heads and phalanges, gradually giving them a "sucked candy cane" appearance (fig. 47).

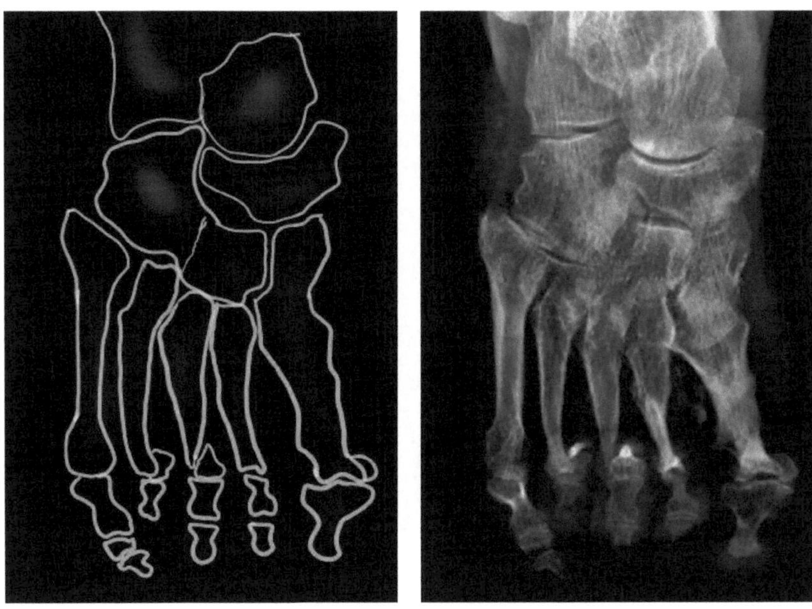

Fig. 47. Nerve osteoarthropathy (a) Diagram. (b) Standard frontal radiograph of the forefoot. Progressive, tapered, sharp-edged osteolysis of the metatarsal heads of the first 4 radii, giving a "candy cane" appearance (arrows). Deforming sequelae of the 4^{e} and 5^{e} metatarsals and misalignment of the metatarsophalangeal joints.

MRI can detect infra-radiological bone signal abnormalities. Subchondral cystic lesions, with a frank T2 hypersignal, are often observed and are highly suggestive diagnostic features [55, 56]. Intra-articular effusion is often observed (fig. 48).

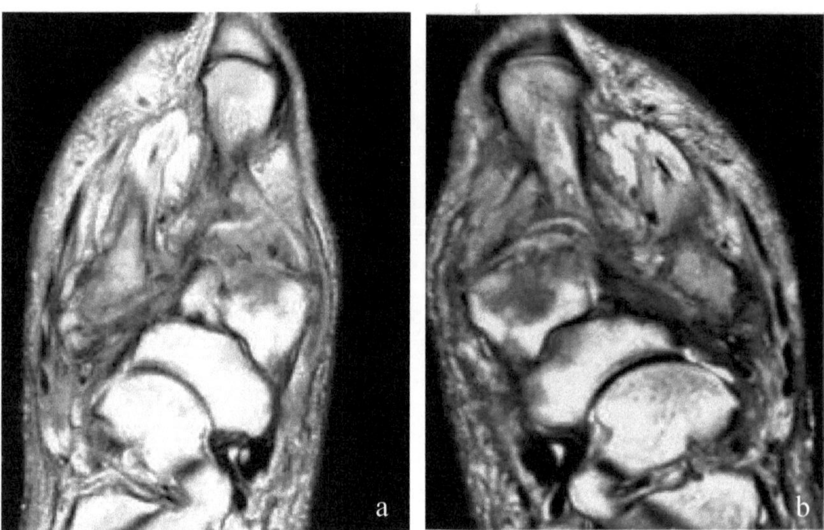

Fig. 48. Nerve osteoarthropathy. MRI (a+b) T2-weighted sequences. (a) T2 hypersignal of subchondral bone (arrow). (b) Intra-articular T2 hypersignal (arrow).

5.1.1.2.Infectious osteoarthropathy

Standard X-rays in infectious osteoarthropathies are indicated in cases of clinical suspicion of new or recurrent infection, plantar perforation disease, for follow-up and comparative imaging.

In the early stages, the standard X-ray may be normal, showing only soft tissue swelling or skin ulceration corresponding to plantar perforator disease (Fig. 49). In the late stage, signs of osteomyelitis may be found, in the form of blurred, poorly limited cortical osteolysis in contact with a wound or area of hyperpressure, with or without a periosteal reaction or bone sequestration (fig. 50). In the case of osteoarthritis, marginal erosions in contact with the skin lesion are highly suggestive (fig. 51).

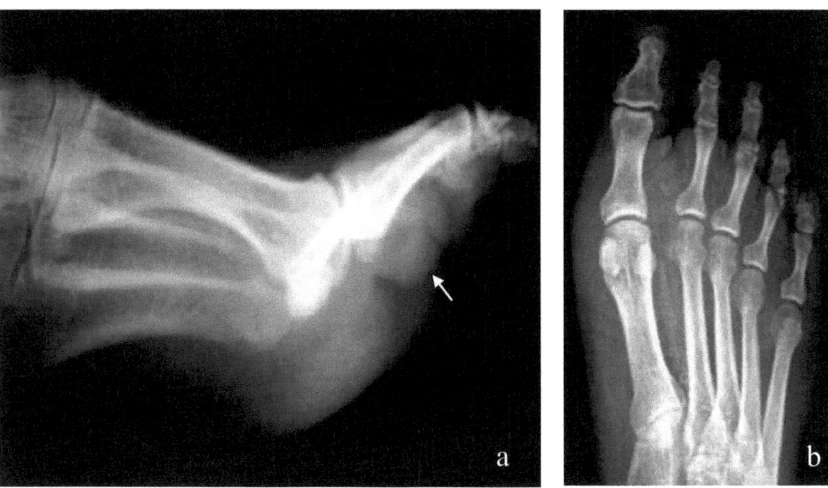

Fig. 49. Infectious osteoarthropathy (a) Standard radiograph of the forefoot in profile. (b) Standard radiograph of the forefoot in profile. (a) Plantar soft tissue swelling (arrow). (b) No bone lesion.

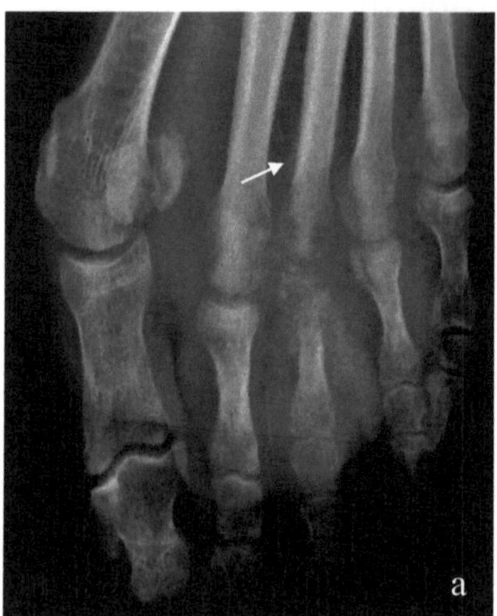

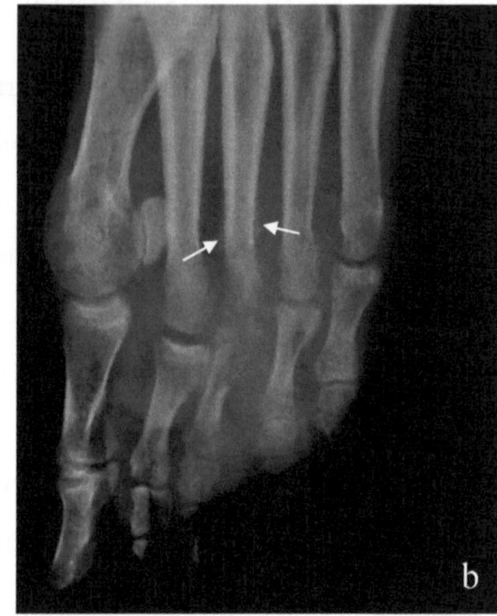

Fig. 50. Infectious osteoarthropathy. (a) Standard radiograph of the forefoot, front. (b) Standard radiograph of the forefoot 3/4. Infectious osteitis of the distal metatarsal and proximal phalanx of the 3^{e} radius of the foot. Bone rarefaction, with blurred contours, associated with a bone periosteal reaction (arrow).

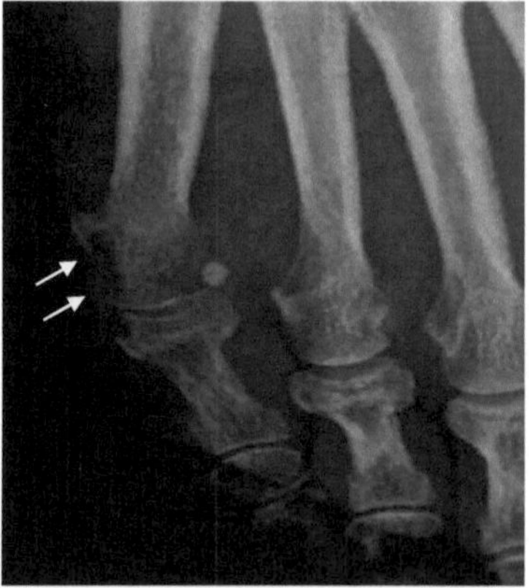

Fig. 51. Infectious osteoarthropathy. Standard radiograph of the front forefoot. Infectious metatarsophangeal osteoarthritis of the 5^{e} radius of the foot. Juxta-articular bone erosions on the lateral side of the joint opposite the skin defect (arrow) [6].

MRI is the gold standard for detecting bone infection. This technique is indicated whenever infection is suspected. T2 STIR is the reference sequence.

It shows bone edema in hyposignal T1 and hypersignal T2, intensely enhanced after injection of contrast medium (fig. 52). Cellulitis may be observed, presenting as soft tissue infiltration with T1 hyposignal and T2 hypersignal, enhancing after contrast; ulceration or fistula, corresponding to loss of substance with empty T1 and T2 signal due to gas artefacts. Inflammation may extend to tendon structures, leading to tenosynovitis, or to the joint, manifested by intra-articular effusion and edema of the margins, or soft-tissue fluid collection (abscess).

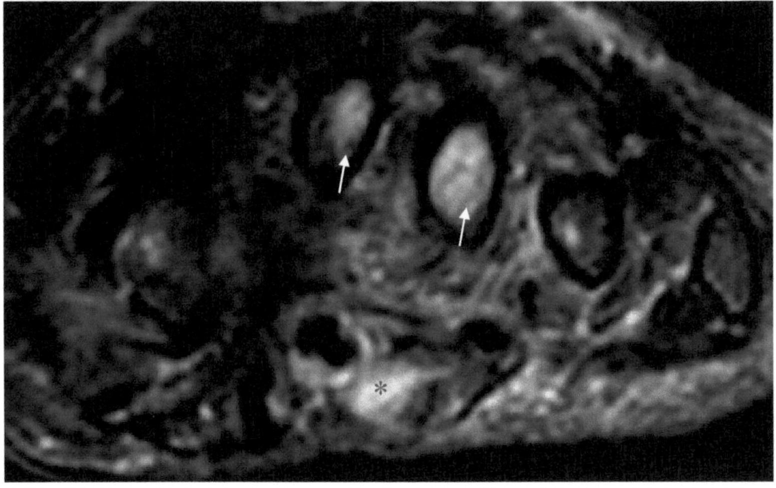

Fig. 52. Infectious osteoarthropathy. MRI, T2-weighted STIR sequence of the forefoot. Hypersignal bone edema (arrow). Soft tissue fluid infiltration predominantly intertendinous (asterisk).

6. Gonads

Regulation of sex hormone secretion is under the control of the hypothalamohypophyseal axis. Gonadotropin-releasing hormone (GnRH), secreted by the hypothalamus, influences pituitary secretion of the gonadotropins follicle-stimulating hormone (FSH) and luteinizing hormone (LH). These act on the
gonads to stimulate secretion of the sex hormones estrogen and progesterone in women and testosterone in men.
FSH has a direct effect on bone metabolism, modulating osteoclast activity and thus promoting bone remodelling. However, estrogen and testosterone have an anabolic effect on bone tissue, acting directly on bone cells [57].

6.1. Hypergonadism

Hypergonadism is responsible for precocious puberty in children and its consequences on bone tissue. The etiologies are multiple, idiopathic or secondary to brain tumors, phacomatoses etc... The secretion of sex hormones stimulates growth, but also bone maturation. Bone age is thus in advance of civil and statural age (fig. 53).

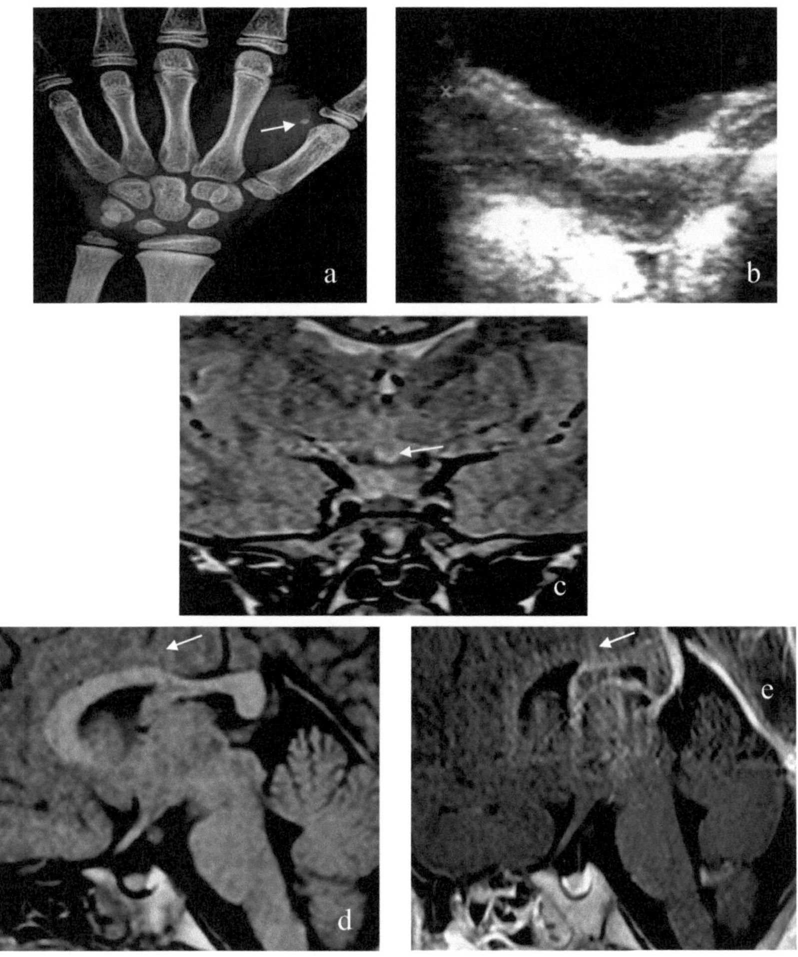

Fig. 53. Hypergonadism. Girl, 4 years old, consulted for precocious puberty and increased LH and FSH levels (a) Standard radiographs of the hand from the front. Bone age 11 years, appearance of thumb sesamoid bone (arrow). (b) Pelvic ultrasound. Pubertal uterus with pyriform appearance. (c) MRI, T2-weighted sequence. (d) MRI, T1-weighted sequence. (e) MRI, T1-weighted sequence after injection of contrast medium. Rounded, well-limited mass, appended to the mammillary tubercles, isosignal to the T1 brain parenchyma, discreetly hypersignal T2, unenhanced (arrow), corresponds to tuber cinereum hamartoma.

6.2. Hypogonadism

Hypogonadism is a deficiency of sex hormones. The consequences of this deficiency on the musculoskeletal system vary according to age.

In children, the etiologies of hypogonadism are generally congenital, secondary to gonadal dysgenesis in Klinefelter's syndrome in boys and Turner's syndrome in girls. In Turner syndrome, estrogen deficiency is also responsible for delayed growth and bone maturation, as measured by bone age. In Klinefelter's syndrome, subjects are tall, mainly due to excessive growth of the lower limbs, with an increased risk of epiphysiolysis [58].

In adults, the radiological sign of hypogonadism is osteoporosis. Today, the radiological diagnosis of osteoporosis is based on the estimation of bone mineral density using two-photon X-ray absorptiometry (osteodensitometry).

The radiological anomalies of osteoporosis are :

- Rarefaction of horizontal trabecular bone trabeculae.
- Preservation of the vertical trabeculae and cortical bone of the vertebral end plates (fig. 54).
- Empty vertebrae or "ghosts".
- Wedge-shaped deformation of the vertebral bodies (fig. 55).
- Staggered vertebral compression (fig. 56).

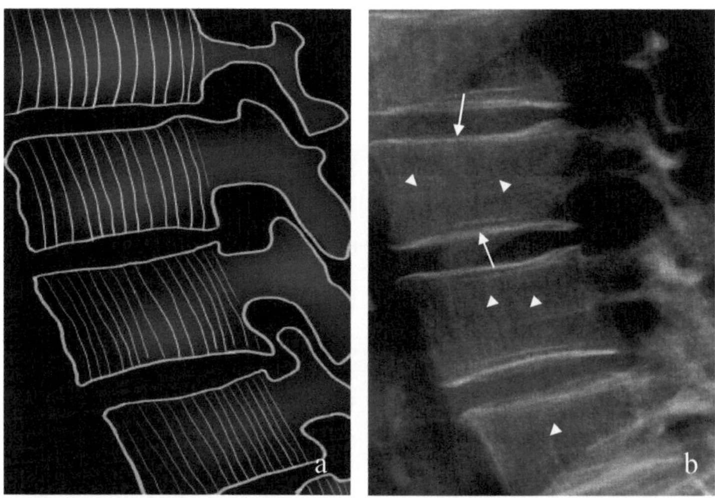

Fig. 54. Osteoporosis (a) Diagram. (b) Standard spine radiograph in profile. Hypertransparency and demineralization of cancellous bone of vertebral bodies contrasting with dense appearance of plateaus (arrows). Preservation of vertical trabeculae (arrowheads).

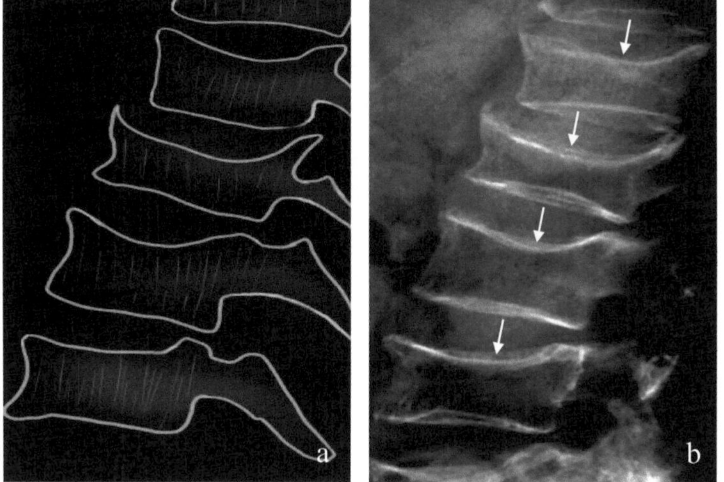

Fig. 55. Osteoporosis (a) Diagram. (b) Standard spine radiograph in profile. Bone demineralization, wedge-shaped and biconcave vertebral settlements (arrows).

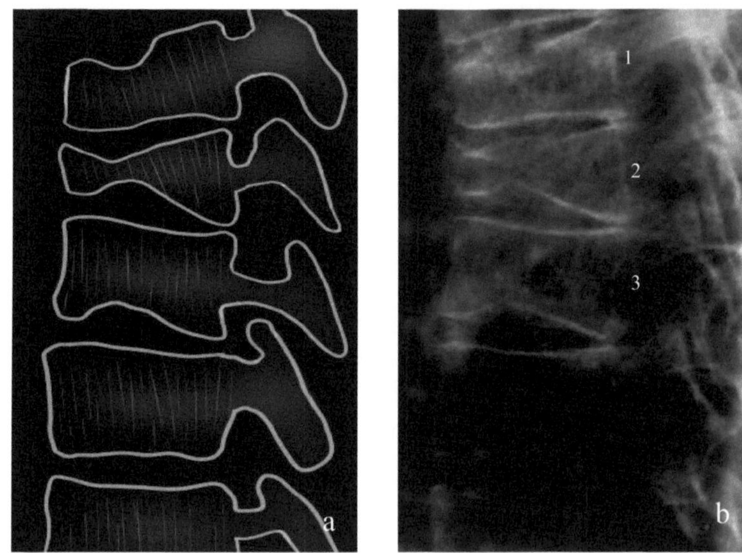

Fig. 56. Osteoporosis (a) Diagram. (b) Standard spine radiograph in profile. Bone demineralization, staggered vertebral settlements. 1. Trapezoidal compression. 2. Complete vertebral compression, vertebra plana. 3. Cupuliform deformation of the vertebral plateau.

References

1. WangY, Nishida S, Elalieh HZ, Long RK, Halloran BP, Bikle DD. Role of IGF-I signaling in regulating osteoclastogenesis. J Bone Miner Res 2006;21:1350-8.
2. Rosen CJ, Motyl KJ. No bones about it: insulin modulates skeletal remodeling. Cell 2010;142:198-200.
3. Chanson P, Salenave S. Acromegaly. Orphanet J Rare Dis 2008;3: 17.
4. Herbinet P, MusielakZanetti C, Chabi N, Cortet B, Cotten A, Endocrinopathies. In: Cotten A, editor. Imagerie musculosquelettique : pathologies générales. Paris : Elsevier-Masson; 2005.p.139-69.
5. Dworakowska D, Gueorguiev M, Kelly P, Monson JP, Besser GM, Chew SL, et al. Repeated colonoscopic screening of patients with acromegaly: 15-year experience identifies those at risk of new colonic neoplasia and allows for effective screening guidelines. Eur J Endocrinol 2010;163:21-8.
6. Lambert A., Loffroy R., Feydy A., Thévenin F., Merzoug V., Méjean N., Couaillier J.-F., Barral F.-G., Chevrot A., Drapé J.-L., Krausé D. Osteoarthropathies of endocrine origin. EMC (Elsevier Masson SAS, Paris), Radiology and medical imaging -musculoskeletal - neurological - maxillofacial, 31-175-B-10, 20111.
7. TaniY, Tanaka N, Isoya E. Locking of metacarpophalangeal joints in a patient with acromegaly. Skeletal Radiol 1999; 28:655-7.
8. obs. UCL Pr A van de Berg, J Malghem
9. Singh GR, Menon PS. Pachydermoperiostosis in a 13 year-old boy presenting as an acromegaly-like syndrome. J Pediatr Endocrinol Metab 1995;8:51-4.
10. Wüster C, Abs R, Bengtsson BA, Bennmarker H, Feldt-Rasmussen U, Hernberg-Ståhl E, et al. The influence of growth hormone deficiency,

growth hormone replacement therapy, and other aspects of hypopituitarism on fracture rate and bone mineral density. J Bone Miner Res 2001;16:398-405.

11. Puel O, Dufillot D, Guillard JM. Hip diseases and growth hormone deficiency. Arch Fr Pediatr 1992;49:437-9.
12. de Andrade AC, Longui CA, Damasceno FL, Santili C. Southwick's angle determination during growth hormone treatment and its usefulness to evaluate risk of epiphysiolysis. J Pediatr Orthop B 2009; 18:11-5.
13. Doga M, Bonadonna S, Gola M, Mazziotti G, Nuzzo M, GiustinaA.GH deficiency in the adult and bone. J Endocrinol Invest 2005;28:18-23.
14. Di Somma C, Colao A, Di Sarno A. Bone marker and bone density responses to dopamine agonist therapy in hyperprolactinemic males. J Clin Endocrinol Metab 1998;83:807-13.
15. Vignali E, Viccica G, Diacinti D. Morphometric vertebral fractures in postmenopausal women with primary hyperparathyroidism. J Clin Endocrinol Metab 2009;94:2306-12.
16. Miller BS, Dimick J, Wainess R, Burney RE. Age- and sex-related incidence of surgically treated primary hyperparathyroidism. World J Surg. 2008 May;32(5):795-9.
17. Aliyev A, Kabasakal L, Simsek O, Paksoy M, Halac M, Uslu I. Ectopic parathyroid adenoma localized with MIBI scintigraphy and excised with guide of macroaggregated human serum albumin injection. Clin Nucl Med 2010;35:151-3.
18. Herbinet P, Musielak-Zanetti C, Chabi N, Cortet B, Cotten A. Endocrinopathies. In: CottenA, editor. Imagerie musculosquelettique: pathologies générales. Paris: Elsevier-Masson; 2005. p. 139-69.
19. Knowles NG, Smith DL, Outwater EK. MRI diagnosis of brown tumor based on magnetic susceptibility. J Magn Reson Imaging 2008;28: 759-61.

20. Hong WS, Sung MS, Chun KA, Kim JY, Park SW, Lee KH, et al. Emphasis on the MR imaging findings of brown tumor: a report of five cases. Skeletal Radiol 2010;Jun13
21. Dussault RG, Kaplan PA. Bone Metabolism Disorders. Endocrine Osteopathies. In: Laredo JD, Morvan G, Wybier M, editors. Imagerie Ostéo-Articulaire. Pathologies générales. Paris: Flammarion; 1998. p. 27-37.
22. Jouan A, Zabraniecki L, Vincent V, Poix E, Fournie B. An unusual presentation of primary hyperparathyroidism: severe hypercalcemia and multiple brown tumors. Joint Bone Spine 2008;75:209-11.
23. Diamanti-Kandarakis E, Livadas S, Tseleni-Balafouta S. Brown tumor of the fibula: unusual presentation of an uncommon manifestation. Report of a case and review of the literature. Endocrine 2007;32: 345-9.
24. DaviesAM,Evans N, Mangham DC, Grimer RJ.MRimaging of brown tumour with fluid-fluid levels: a report of three cases. Eur Radiol 2001; 11:1445-9.
25. Rubin MR, Silverberg SJ. Rheumatic manifestations of primary hyperparathyroidism and parathyroid hormone therapy. Curr Rheumatol Rep 2002;4:179-85.
26. Maeda SS, Fortes EM, Oliveira UM, Borba VC, Lazaretti-Castro M. Hypoparathyroidism and pseudohypoparathyroidism. Arq Bras Endocrinol Metabol 2006;50:664-73.
27. Bindu M, Harinarayana CV. Hypoparathyroidism: a rare treatable cause of epilepsy - report of two cases. Eur J Neurol 2006;13:786-8.
28. Rubin MR, Dempster DW, Kohler T. Three dimensional cancellous bone structure in hypoparathyroidism. Bone 2010;46:190-5.
29. Rubin MR, Dempster DW, Zhou H, Shane E, Nickolas T, Sliney Jr. J, et al. Dynamic and structural properties of the skeleton in hypoparathyroidism. J Bone Miner Res 2008;23:2018-24.

30.Unverdi S, Ozturk MA, Inal S. Idiopathic hypoparathyroidism mimicking diffuse idiopathic skeletal hyperostosis. J Clin Rheumatol 2009;15:361-2.
31.Mamdani N, Repp AL, Seyoum B, Berhanu P. Idiopathic hypoparathyroidism presenting with severe hypocalcemia and asymptomatic basal ganglia calcification followed by acute intracerebral bleed. Endocr Pract 2007;13:487-92.
32.Vestergaard P, Mosekilde L. Hyperthyroidism, bone mineral, and fracture risk--a meta-analysis. Thyroid 2003;13:585-93.
33.Batal O, Hatem SF. Radiologic case study. Thyroid acropachy. Orthopedics 2008;31(2):98-100.
34.FatourechiV,Ahmed DD, Schwartz KM. Thyroid acropachy: report of 40 patients treated at a single institution in a 26-year period. J Clin Endocrinol Metab 2002;87:5435-41.
35.Simic N, Asztalos EV, Rovet J. Impact of neonatal thyroid hormone insufficiency and medical morbidity on infant neurodevelopment and attention following preterm birth. Thyroid 2009;19:395-401.
36.Gruters A, Krude H. Update on the management of congenital hypothyroidism. Horm Res 2007;68(suppl5):107-11.
37.Vestergaard P,Weeke J, Hoeck HC. Fractures in patients with primary idiopathic hypothyroidism. Thyroid 2000;10:335-40.
38.Vestergaard P, Mosekilde L. Fractures in patients with hyperthyroidismand hypothyroidism: a nationwide follow-up study in 16,249 patients. Thyroid 2002;12:411-9.
39.Lodish MB, Hsiao HP, Serbis A, Sinaii N, Rothenbuhler A, Keil MF, et al. Effects of Cushing disease on bone mineral density in a pediatric population. J Pediatr 2010;156:1001-5.
40.Chiodini I, MorelliV, Masserini B. Bone mineral density, prevalence of vertebral fractures, and bone quality in patients with adrenal

incidentalomas with and without subclinical hypercortisolism: an Italian multicenter study. J Clin Endocrinol Metab 2009;94: 3207-14.

41. Chiodini I, Torlontano M, Carnevale V, Trischitta V, Scillitani A. Skeletal involvement in adult patients with endogenous hypercortisolism. J Endocrinol Invest 2008;31:267-76.

42. Khanine V, Fournier JJ, Requeda E, Luton JP, Simon F, Crouzet J. Osteoporotic fractures at presentation of Cushing's disease: two case reports and a literature review. Joint Bone Spine 2000;67:341-5.

43. Takada J, Nagoya S, Kuwabara H, Kaya M, Yamashita T. Rapidly destructive coxarthropathy with osteonecrosis and osteoporosis caused by Cushing's syndrome. Orthopedics 2004;27:1111-3.

44. Koch CA, Tsigos C, Patronas NJ, Papanicolaou DA. Cushing's disease presenting with avascular necrosis of the hip: an orthopedic emergency. J Clin Endocrinol Metab 1999;84:3010-2.

45. Hayes CW, Conway WF, Daniel WW. MR imaging of bone marrow edema pattern: transient osteoporosis, transient bone marrow edema syndrome, or osteonecrosis. Radiographics 1993;13:1001-11

46. Vande Berg BE, Malghem JJ, Labaisse MA, Noel HM, Maldague BE. MR imaging of avascular necrosis and transient marrow edema of the femoral head. Radiographics 1993;13:501-20.

47. Dumont-Fischer D, Rat AC. Saidenberg-Kermanac'h N, Laurent S, Cohen R, Boissier MC. Spinal epidural lipomatosis revealing endogenous Cushing's syndrome. Joint Bone Spine 2002;69:222-5.

48. Lopez-Gonzalez A, Resurreccion Giner M. Idiopathic spinal epidural lipomatosis: urgent decompression in an atypical case. Eur Spine J 2008;17(suppl2):S225-S227.

49. Gill JB. Fat suppression imaging in epidural lipomatosis: case report. J Surg Orthop Adv 2007;16:144-7.

50.Montoriol PF, Da Ines D, Bailly A, Garcier JM. Steroid-induced epidural lipomatosis in a patient with sarcoidosis. J Radiol 2010;91: 511-3.

51.Marcus CD, Ladam-Marcus VJ, Leone J, Malgrange D, Bonnet-Gausserand FM, Menanteau BP. MR imaging of osteomyelitis and neuropathic osteoarthropathy in the feet of diabetics. Radiographics 1996;16:1337-48.

52. Schaper NC, Apelqvist J, Bakker K. The international consensus and practical guidelines on the management and prevention of the diabetic foot. Curr Diab Rep 2003;3:475-9.

53.Larroque G, Kamba C, Blin D, Lopez FM, Cyteval C. Imaging of the diabetic foot. J Radiol 2006;87:541-7.

54.Sella EJ, Barrette C. Staging of Charcot neuroarthropathy along the medial column of the foot in the diabetic patient. J Foot Ankle Surg 1999;38:34-40.

55.Schlossbauer T, Mioc T, Sommerey S, Kessler SB, Reiser MF, Pfeifer KJ. Magnetic resonance imaging in early stage Charcot arthropathy: correlation of imaging findings and clinical symptoms. Eur J Med Res 2008;13:409-14.

56.Ahmadi ME, Morrison WB, Carrino JA, Schweitzer ME, Raikin SM, Ledermann HP. Neuropathic arthropathy of the foot with and without superimposed osteomyelitis: MR imaging characteristics. Radiology 2006;238:622-31.

57.Ernst M, Heath JK, Schmid C, Froesch RE, Rodan GA. Evidence for a direct effect of estrogen on bone cells in vitro. J Steroid Biochem 1989; 34:279-84.

58.Primiano GA, Hughston JC. Slipped capital femoral epiphysis in a true hypogonadal male (Klinefelter's mosaic XY-XXY). A case report. J Bone Joint Surg Am 1971;53:597-601.

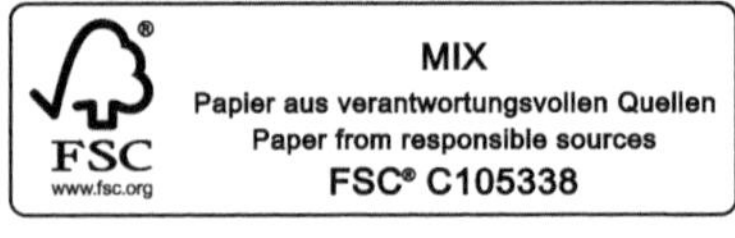

Printed by Books on Demand GmbH, Norderstedt / Germany